CLINICAL CARDIOLOGY

and Electrocardiography

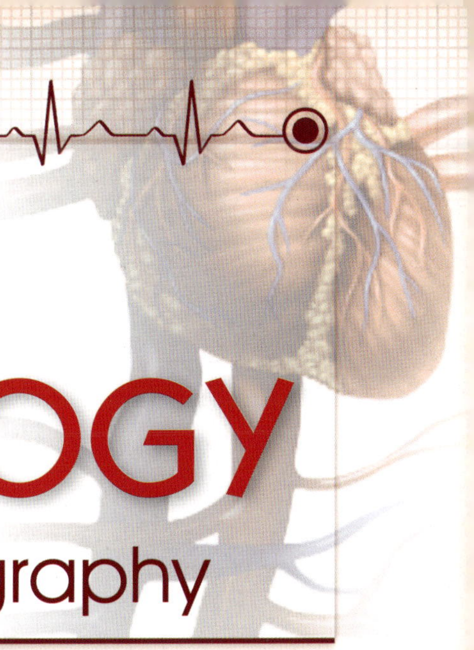

History-Taking, General Physical Examination (Cardiology Related) and Cardiac Examination

CLINICAL CARDIOLOGY

and Electrocardiography

History-Taking, General Physical Examination (Cardiology Related) and Cardiac Examination

BS Cheema VSM

MD (Medicine) DM (Cardiology) FACC (USA) FICC FICP

Formerly

Senior Adviser (Medicine and Cardiology)
AH R & R, Delhi Cantt
Professor, Department of Medicine and
Senior Consultant Cardiologist
KMC, Mangalore and KMC, Manipal
SGRD Medical College, Amritsar
Senior Consultant Cardiologist
MM University Hospital, Mullana (Haryana)

Assisted by

Munish Sharma

MBBS MD (Medicine) DNB (Cardiology)

Associate Professor
Department of Medicine and Cardiology
Command Hospital (WC), Chandimandir

CBSPD

CBS Publishers & Distributors Pvt Ltd

New Delhi • Bengaluru • Chennai • Kochi • Kolkata • Lucknow • Mumbai
Hyderabad • Jharkhand • Nagpur • Patna • Pune • Uttarakhand

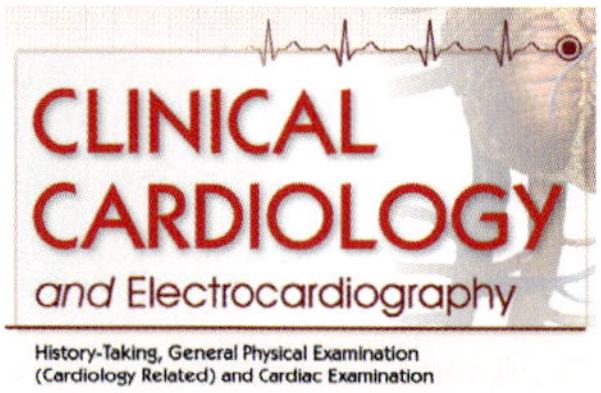

ISBN: 978-93-5466-736-7

First Edition: 2024

Published by Satish Kumar Jain and produced by Varun Jain for
CBS Publishers & Distributors Pvt Ltd
4819/XI Prahlad Street, 24 Ansari Road, Daryaganj, New Delhi 110 002, India
Ph: 011-23289259, 23266861 Website: www.cbspd.com
e-mail: delhi@cbspd.com

Corporate Office: 204 FIE, Industrial Area, Patparganj, Delhi 110 092, India
Ph: 011-49344934 Fax: 011-49344935 e-mail: publishing@cbspd.com; publicity@cbspd.com

Branches

- **Bengaluru:** Seema House 2975, 17th Cross, K.R. Road, Banasankari 2nd Stage, Bengaluru 560 070, Karnataka, India
  Ph: +91-80-26771678/79 Fax: +91-80-26771680 e-mail: bangalore@cbspd.com
- **Chennai:** 7, Subbaraya Street, Shenoy Nagar, Chennai 600 030, Tamil Nadu, India
  Ph: +91-44-26680620, 26681266 Fax: +91-44-42032115 e-mail: chennai@cbspd.com
- **Kochi:** 42/1325, 1326, Power House Road, Opposite KSEB, Power House, Ernakulam 682018, Kochi, Kerala, India
  Ph: +91-484-4059061–65 Fax: +91-484-4059065 e-mail: kochi@cbspd.com
- **Kolkata:** 147, Hind Ceramics Compound, 1st Floor, Nilgunj Road, Belghoria, Kolkata 700056, West Bengal, India
  Ph: +91-33-25330055/56 e-mail: kolkata@cbspd.com
- **Lucknow:** Basement, Khushnuma Complex, 7 Meerabai Marg (behind Jawahar Bhawan), Lucknow 226001, UP, India
  Ph: +91-522-4000032 e-mail: tiwari.lucknow@cbspd.com
- **Mumbai:** PWD Shed, Gala No. 25/26, Ramchandra Bhatt Marg, Next JJ Hospital Gate No. 2, Opp. Union Bank of India, Noorbaug, Mumbai 400009, Maharashtra, India
  Ph: +91-22-66661880/89 e-mail: mumbai@cbspd.com

Representatives

• **Hyderabad**	0-9885175004	• **Jharkhand**	0-9811541605	• **Nagpur**	0-8692091830
• **Patna**	0-9334159340	• **Pune**	0-9664372571	• **Uttarakhand**	0-9716462459

Printed at HT Media Ltd. Greater Noida, UP, India

Preface

This book *Clinical Cardiology with Electrocardiography* covers history, physical exam of heart and ECG examination of common clinical cardiac problems including IHD & ECG related emergencies. I had planned long time back to write this book in clinical cardiology, incorporating my long cardiology teaching experience of about 27 years at different medical colleges and universities in India. It will be useful bedside guide for MD (Med), residents and cardiology residents in their initial part of their training.

ECG recording is a bedside procedure which is done for almost all cardiology cases and relevant medical cases in daily practice in hospitals and private clinic's in India. Correct interpretation of ECG is important for all young and old physicians and cardiologists. After final retirement 4 years back, when I settled in Tricity Chandigarh, I was fortunate to develop a professional contact with Col Munish Sharma, a young brilliant clinical and interventional cardiologist at Command Hospital (WC), Chandimandir. I am also thankful to Col PS Monga, senior adviser (Medicine and Cardiology) for providing me ECGs of complicated cardiac cases as and when required. So taking advantage of my long association with clinical cardiology, and Col Munish' s assistance, I wrote this book of clinical cardiology incorporating ECG examination. The practical management of common cardiac especially ECG related emergencies is discussed in rather detail for the benefit of medicine and cardiology residents so that they diagnose common cardiac problems adapting correct logical and scientific approach to diagnose and treat the patients in minimum time. Thereby we will able to save a lot of cardiac patients.

I am thankful to my daughter Col Sumeet Cheema, a Paediatrician in AMC and my son Dr Mandeep Cheema MD, Professor of Medicine at MM Medical College and Hospital, Solan, who gave me all encouragement for writing this book. My young smart granddaughter Simran, a graduate student at Chandigarh University, was very helpful in making line drawing of pictures whenever required.

Dr Munish Sharma was very helpful in giving me intelligent suggestions in selecting ECG s for presentation in this book. I am ever grateful to him for this help. I also thankful to my part time office staff Mr Rahul Gulati and Miss Maninderjit Kaur for all the clerical job besides writing and labeling the pictures to make this book in presentable form in stipulated time.

I am thankful to CBS Publishers & Distributers Pvt Ltd, especially Mr YN Arjuna and Mr SK Verma, for accepting my book for publication, I will be ever grateful to them.

BS Cheema VSM
Senior Consultant Cardiologist

Contents

Clinical Examination of Heart and Cardiovascular System

Introduction

Thorough history taking along with clinical examination in present time is as mandatory as it was in previous years since long back. We can get many useful clues directing us to correct diagnosis of cardiac and peripheral vascular disease, besides many electronic and computer-based modern diagnostic aids being available in the modern cardiology and medicine practice. The medical students should master art of good history taking and clinical examination as is being elaborated in this document.

As the patient walks into clinic or cardiac OPD room, his gait besides built is assessed. **For example: Hemiplegic** gait suggestive of CVA is most usually associated with hypertension, or stooping, posture with shuffling, short stepping gait and tremors of the hands point to **parkinsonism**. Patient may come in a wheel chair, either being too old to walk or due to multiple disabilities, advanced CCF, or severe chest pain of myocardial infarction. All these patients should be seen on priority, as an octogenarian patient with multiple disabilities. The young medicos and the junior medical staff must be taught to be respectful and helpful to senior citizens as is our oriental culture.

In the medical history related to cardiology important symptoms should be asked to the patient even by leading questions if he/she has not mentioned it, as detailed in Chapter 1 of this document.

Section

1

Physical Examination

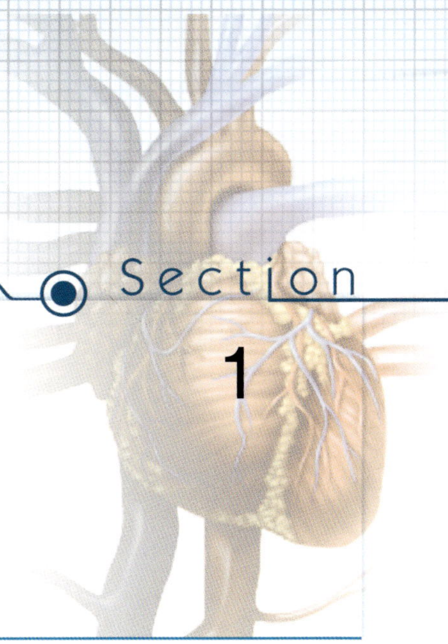

1. History of Present Illness
2. General Physical Examination: Clues to Cardiac Disease
3. Blood Pressure Evaluation
4. Examination of Heart

Chapter 1

History of Present Illness

Time spent in talking to a patient is valuable in getting important first-hand information about his/her illness besides establishing a long-term bond of mutual trust and confidence with the patient.

The most important symptoms of cardiac illness are:

(a) **Dyspnoea**, (b) **Chest pain**, (c) **Syncope**, (d) **Palpitation**, (e) **Oedema**, (f) **Fatigue**, (g) **Fever**, (h) **Claudication on walking**. In history, we also evaluate patient's **dietary habits** and **type of lifestyle** and any **drug intake besides past illness**, if any.

DYSPNOEA

It means difficulty in breathing. It is an abnormal uncomfortable awareness of self-breathing.

Common causes are cardiac and respiratory diseases. Dyspnoea can develop suddenly/acutely or can be of gradual onset with progression.

Causes of Acute Sudden Dyspnoea

a. Cardiac causes

1. Acute pulmonary oedema–acute LVF (left ventricular failure)
2. Acute pulmonary embolism.

b. Respiratory causes

1. Pneumothorax
2. Bronchopneumonia
3. Acute airway obstruction.

Special Type of Acute Dyspnoea

PND (Paroxysmal Nocturnal Dyspnoea)

A classical symptom of LVF: A known cardiac patient usually sleeps with pillows at back, with sleep, he slips down and lies flat, then he wakes up suddenly mostly after midnight with sudden breathing difficulty, gasping for breath, sweating with mild wheezing followed by cough, after he gets up he feels better in 10–20 minutes.

Pathogenesis

1. On change of posture, venous return to lungs increases. It causes pulmonary congestion in an already congested lungs and stimulation of Hering-Breuer stretch receptors of alveoli causes sudden stimulation of depressed respiratory centre leading to episodes of hyperpnoea.

2. **Increased stimulation of sympathetic activity that occurs** in the period of REM sleep at the central level in the medulla. These two factors increase the respiratory rate and patient becomes dyspnoeic. On change of posture, pulmonary congestion becomes less and the breathing becomes better.

Differential diagnosis: Acute bronchial asthma—**status asthmaticus**. In this cough is earlier, dyspnoea later and symptoms take hours to be relieved.

Chronic Progressive Dyspnoea

It is due to slowly developing pulmonary congestion and interstitial oedema in lungs in long-standing left heart disease cases.

NYHA (New York Heart Association) functional classification of dyspnoea or effort intolerance is **internationally** accepted (Table 1.1).

Table 1.1: NYHA classification of patients with cardiac disease

Class I	No limitation on physical activity in ordinary work, but he/she cannot compete in strenuous work with healthy persons of the same age and sex.
Class II	Slight limitation of physical activity, on ordinary work gets fatigue and dyspnoea. Cannot climb 1st floor of a house without dyspnoea.
Class III	Dyspnoea on less than ordinary physical activity, comfortable at rest. Patient gets dyspnoeic on household walking like going to the bathroom, etc.
Class IV	Dyspnoea on rest; cannot perform any activity without dyspnoea and sits in his/her bed even during daytime.

Types of Dyspnoea

1. **Orthopnoea:** Symptom of LVF. Dyspnoea on lying down. Relieved on sitting up.
2. **Trepopnoea:** Dyspnoea on lateral position, e.g. unilateral lung disease.
3. **Platypnoea:** Dyspnoea on sitting up, e.g. left atrial myxoma and orthostatic hypotension.

Common Causes of Chronic Dyspnoea

1. LVF (left ventricular failure)
2. CCF (congestive cardiac failure)
3. COPD (chronic obstructive pulmonary disease)
4. Chronic restrictive lung disease and ILD (interstitial lung disease).

Cough

Less specific symptom in cardiac lesion.

More commonly in COPD and other lung diseases.

In cardiac cases these days, commonest causes are:

1. Patients on ACE inhibitor drugs for the treatment of hypertension, as they activate Bradykinin which stimulates cough centre.
2. PAH (pulmonary arterial hypertension) in severe mitral stenosis (MS), mostly nocturnal cough.

1

Haemoptysis: Blood in sputum (up to 60 ml fresh blood).

Causes: Cardiac
1. Mitral stenosis
2. Acute pulmonary oedema
3. Pulmonary infarction
4. Anticoagulant drug overdose.

Common non-cardiac causes:
1. Pulmonary tuberculosis
2. Bronchogenic carcinoma
3. Pulmonary trauma.

CHEST PAIN

It is a more frequent symptom and difficult to analyse. Classical chest pain due to ischemic heart disease is called **angina pectoris–when there is a discrepancy between demand and supply of oxygen to myocardium**.

Angina pectoris: Classically it is dull pressure type of discomfort, felt as choking sensation or a sense of tightness in the chest. It is not pricking type. Patient may describe it with a fist of the hand placed on the chest wall **(Levine's sign)**. It lasts for a few minutes to 30 minutes and it is precipitated by physical effort or mental stress. It may occur at night or most commonly it occurs in early morning due to increased sympathetic activity. It is relieved by rest and lying down or by tablet Trinitroglycerin S/L (TNG) or on relief of mental tension. This pain radiates to left shoulder and left arm, medial side of forearms, and in medial two fingers of the left hand. Rarely it may start in left hand and move upwards to left shoulder. It sometimes goes to neck and teeth. In ischemia of inferior wall, mild epigastric pain with abdominal distension may be the only symptom pain not felt below umbilicus.

Rarely in advanced ischaemic heart disease (IHD), on lying down due to increased venous return, workload of the heart increases and hence more episodes of angina may occur, relieved on sitting up **(angina decubitus)**.

Angina at Night

1. **Prinzmetal variant angina** due to coronary artery spasm
2. IHD with LVF
3. Severe AS (aortic stenosis) with significant LV outlet obstruction and LVH.

Painless IHD: Seen in cases of—
1. Diabetes mellitus—due to autonomic neuropathy pain is not transmitted to thalamus
2. Old age—due to age-related autonomic neuropathy
3. Cardiac transplant
4. More so in females.

Like dyspnoea, for better scientific communication and documentation, chest pain due to angina pectoris has been functionally classified by the **Canadian Cardiovascular Society**.

Class I	Walking/climbing upstairs upto first floor no chest pain but angina with strenuous/rapid exertion.
Class II	Rapid walking 1–2 km at a lower speed, climbing upto first floor produces angina or under emotional stress.
Class III	Marked limitation of physical effort. Walking on level at a leisure pace for short distances causes pain.
Class IV	Angina at rest.

Recent angina and recurrent angina at rest are called unstable angina.

Angina of recent onset 4–6 weeks, and recurrent angina at rest are called unstable angina and angina over 1 hour mostly due to impending acute myocardial infarction called **acute coronary syndrome (ACS)**.

So causes of acute discomfort in the chest due to IHD are:

1. Stable angina pectoris
2. Unstable angina } ACS
3. Acute myocardial infarction }

Other Cardiac Related Causes of Chest Pain

1. **Acute dissection of aorta**. **Severe chest** pain going to back with diminution of femoral pulses and severe hypotension or severe hypertension.
2. **Acute pericarditis pain** is going to left shoulder, sharp continuous more on lying down, relief on sitting and leaning forward, fever, sweating.
3. **Acute myocarditis** pain and tachycardia, diminished heart sounds ↑S3+ JVP raised.

If **acute MI** (myocardial infarction) is diagnosed by urgent ECG, and if pain does not respond to 3 doses of S/L TNG (trinitroglycerin) given at 15 minutes. Interval with levels of Raised Serum Troponin, showing evidence of muscle necrosis. Such patient of ACS should be sent to the nearest hospital where facilities for thrombolysis are available or for doing coronary angiography and PTCA (stent application) by expert interventional cardiologist. Patient should reach such hospitals in **12 hours** from the onset of chest pain.

Other Common Causes of Chest Pain

1. Pleurisy increasing on coughing + chest signs.
2. **Acute pulmonary embolism:** Bedridden patient suddenly becomes dyspnoeic, in mostly surgical hip operated cases. Moderate chest pain and cyanosis with hypotension + sweating.
3. **Anxiety:** Pricking pain with hyperventilation + serial ECG normal, usually pain stays for hours + sweating.
4. Esophageal spasm and reflux oesophagitis cause abdominal distension.
5. Musculoskeletal pain is relieved with antacids, proton pump inhibitors like pantoprazole, and NSAID analgesic localized tenderness (Tietze syndrome of acute costochondritis).
6. Referred from cervical spine in cervical spondylosis.
7. History of past chest trauma.

SYNCOPE

It is defined as a sudden loss of consciousness.

Sudden loss of consciousness is due to reduced blood supply and reduced perfusion of the brain.

Sudden loss of consciousness without preceding aura or any other symptom is usually due to cardiac cause like:

1. Stokes-Adams AV block sudden transient loss of consciousness upto few seconds
2. LVF
3. LVT
4. Asystole
5. Sick sinus syndrome.

Syncope due to cardiac cause rarely lasts for more than 2–3 minutes, if more than this then, non-cardiac cause.

- Syncope precipitated by effort in PAH (pulmonary arterial hypertension).
- **Family history of syncope—epilepsy**, long QT interval in ECG.
- **Position at onset**—standing → hypotension
- **Relation to food**—hypoglycemia associated sweating.
- **Prolonged standing—vasodepressor syncope** by decreased cardiac output, developing gradually induced by emotional stress autonomic nervous system ↑increased vagal tone, bradycardia. Relieved by lying down–**residual bradycardia**. Common in young Army/Police recruits in TRG (training) centres.
- **Carotid syncope**—hypersensitive carotid sinus pressed by **tight collar in old age. Relieved immediately on removing the tight collar**.
- Postsyncope sign is mostly neurological, e.g. **epilepsy** associated **incontinence of urine**.

PALPITATIONS

- Defined as the unpleasant awareness of forceful or rapid beating of the heart. Careful history will tell us the exact cause.
- **Commonest causes are** anxiety—increase in HR > 140/min, and hyperventilation.
- If isolated jumps or skips in arterial pulse—**extrasystole**.
- If acute onset abruptly with HR> 120/min and abrupt ending—**paroxysmal atrial tachycardia (PAT)**.

Independent of exercise: Thyrotoxicosis, **LVF**, anaemia **Heart rate 120–150/min, AF** (atrial flutter), **PAT**. Excess tea, coffee and alcohol intake cause palpitation.

OEDEMA

- Weight gain of 3–5 kg occurs before oedema develops.
- **Unilateral leg oedema**, caused by—saphenous vein harvesting for CABG, deep vein thrombosis in the lower limb.
- **If ascites precedes oedema—unlikely to be due to heart disease**—causes, cirrhosis of liver, constrictive pericarditis. Oedema, **ascites**, and no LVF-tricuspid regurgitation constrictive pericarditis.

- **Oedema of face, arms, and elevated JVP with no pulsation, superior mediastinal obstruction.**
- **Periorbital oedema—renal causes**
- **Drugs**—calcium channel blockers (amlodipine, diltiazem), long-term use. In hypertension cases and steroid therapy.
- **Generalised anasarca**—unusual in CCF. More in myxoedema and hypoproteinaemia (Fig. 1.1).

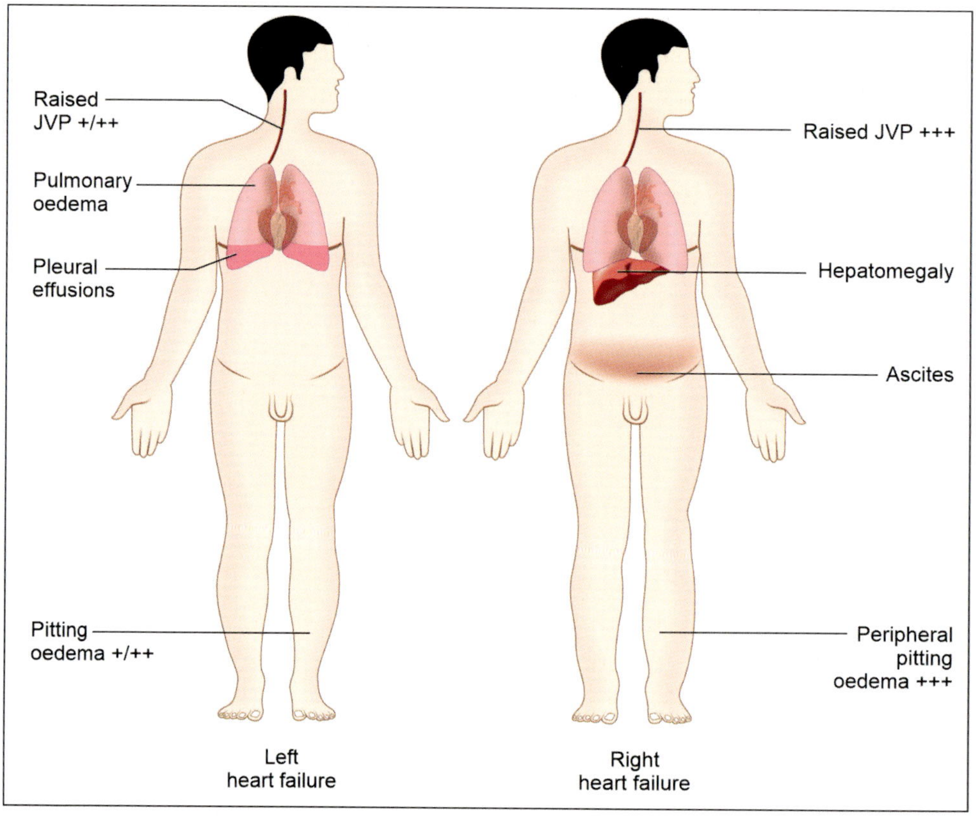

Fig. 1.1

JOINT PAINS

Suggestive of rheumatic fever even mild arthralgia—more common in Indian patients than full-fledged arthritis, arthralgia especially in younger age—acute rheumatic fever, fleeting joint pain.

FEVER

1

Low grade/remittent/continuous fever with a history of heart disease in childhood **congenital heart disease and rheumatic heart disease** is suggestive of infective endocarditis.

History of drug prophylaxis—injection benzathine penicillin dose 1.2 million units once a month in rheumatic heart disease. History of recurrent palpitation with chest infection in childhood suggest L–R Shunt lesion, i.e. **VSD, PDA, ASD**.

Fatigue, common in CCF occurs with low cardiac output. **Drugs like diuretics** and beta blockers. Emotional stress precedes and accompanies acute MI.

History of Past Illness

1. History of diabetes mellitus, hypertension, obesity, and smoking should be checked in each case of IHD and also in close family members as these are risk factors of IHD.
2. **Cardiac murmur** during childhood—VSD, ASD, PDA, rheumatic heart disease.
3. **Cyanosis**—tetralogy of Fallot and other cyanotic congenital heart diseases since birth, e.g. TGA, TAT.
4. **COPD and smoking**—cor pulmonale.
5. **Alcohol**—chronic alcoholic is one consuming more than 150 ml in per day for 5 years. It leads to cardiomyopathy **holiday heart syndrome**, which occurs after acute alcoholism in a young couples competing with each other on beer bottles during honeymoon—acute **AF after an alcoholic binge requires urgent DC conversion**.

Age, Race and Sex

In South Asians: **Truncal obesity and CAD (coronary artery disease)** much earlier between 30 and 40 years of age and more common in both males and females also show high levels of serum triglyceride and insulin resistance.

Rheumatic heart disease: **Incidence is more in developing countries and in** younger age groups. **Juvenile RHD <18 years**.

Age

1. **CHD (congenital heart disease)** since birth atrial septal defect (ASD), ventricular septal defect (VSD), patent ductus arteriosus (PDA), and cyanotic heart diseases, e.g. tetralogy of fallot (TOF), transposition great arteries (TGA), double outlet right ventricle (DORVS), tricuspid atresia with pulmonary stenosis.
2. **Bicuspid aortic valve is commonest in adults**.
3. **Calcific AS (aortic stenosis)** in amyloidosis, mitral annulus calcification more in old age.
4. **IHD in South Asians**—high prevalence after 25 years of age as mentioned earlier/ sex in females and males equal preponderance of IHD in South Asia, unlike Western population, whereas in males it is more than females.
5. ASD/HOCM/IHD/hypertension have a strong family history. In India prevalence **hypertension is 33% (every third person) (now 33.5%, as per latest ICMR report after 12 years follows up)**.
6. **ASD** is more in females.
7. **IHD** is more in males and after 25–35 years.
8. **Mitral stenosis**—in the Indian population equal incidence in males and females. Occurs fully developed after rheumatic fever at juvenile age group <18 years in many children. First described in AIIMS, New Delhi in 1960.
9. **Diet**—vegetarian/non-vegetarian—obesity, which cooking oil used—desi ghee/olive oil/saffola oil/Sunola oil/rice bran oil/mustard oil for cooking. Using mustard oil for long time can cause complete heart block.

FAMILY HISTORY

ASD, HOCM, IHD, hypertension and PAH runs in families, more familial predisposition. Hypertension is a commonest human disease in developed and developing countries. So also in India, it is commonest disease (33.5% prevalence). In Punjab, every second person is having hypertension especially with truncal obesity and diabetes mellitus.

INTERMITTENT CLAUDICATION

Patients who are chainsmokers (more than 10 cigarettes per day for over 5 years), develop either Buerger's disease or peripheral arterial atherosclerosis. These patients after walking for a short distance of 1–2 km get pain in the legs. On taking rest this pain is relieved. Peripheral atherosclerosis is as common as coronary or cerebral atherosclerosis.

In such cases, all peripheral arterial pulsations—both brachialis, radials, femorals, posttibials, and dorsalis pedis, should be felt. Any sign of impending gangrene is to be noted at any limb. If history of renal disease with hypertension, then area over both renal arteries in paraumbilical region of the abdomen, must be auscultated for renal bruits of renal artery stenosis.

Chapter 2

General Physical Examination: Clues to Cardiac Disease

GENERAL BODY BUILT

1. **Unusually tall individuals**

   Marfan's syndrome

   i. Arm span > height
   ii. Lower segment (pubis-foot) is longer than upper segment
   iii. Arachnodactyly
   iv. Ectopia lentis
   v. Thumb sign-protrusion of thumb beyond folded fingers in hand.

   With an **X-ray of the hand-metacarpal index**—ratio of length of the five metacarpal bones to width is between 5.6 and 7.5. More than 8.5 in Marfan syndrome.

   Marfan's syndrome is associated with **MVP (mitral valve prolapse), AR (aortic regurgitation), MR (mitral regurgitation), aortic root dilation and aortic aneurysm.**
2. **Kyphoscoliosis:** Leads to advanced cor pulmonale.
3. **Pectus excavatum** with a straight back supine. Take an X-ray lateral view of the chest—measure distance between vertebral column and posterior sternum at the level of the 4th dorsal vertebra. Normal is 6 cm.

   Mild and moderate: If 5 cm or more.

   Severe: If <5 cm.

Cardiac Conditions Associated with Pectus Excavatum

a. **MVP (mitral valve prolapse)**
b. Cardiac compression pseudo heart disease–pancake heart on X-ray chest AP view.
c. **Benign systolic murmur at the pulmonary area.**

Obesity is Defined when:

a. **Body mass index (BMI)**, i.e. ratio of weight in kg/height in m^2 is **more than 25 in Indians.**
b. **Waist/hip ratio**, i.e. diameter of waist/diameter of hip, is >0.85; normal is up to 0.8, if more than 0.8 then trunkal obesity is seen in South Asians and is associated with hypertension, hypertriglyceridemia, hyperinsulinaemia and IHD between 25 years and 40 years.
c. **Obesity** is a risk factor for **IHD, hypertension, and diabetes mellitus.**

d. **Obesity (gross) cause of:**
   i. Sleep apnoea syndrome
   ii. Cardiomyopathy
   iii. Oedema of feet.

PHYSICAL APPEARANCES

1. Hemiplegic gait due to an old CVA in a known case of hypertension/cardiac lesion (valvular, post-MI) source of **mural thrombus in LA**.
2. Hyperthyroidism—anxious, exophthalmos.
3. **Neurocirculatory asthenia**—a tense, anxious young individual palmar sweating, sighing respiration, tachycardia and pricking chest pain–may be hyperventilating. Seen in anxiety state, especially in young army and police recruits/workers who want to avoid work and feign cardiac illness.

Body Posture

1. Acutely ill patient with rapid breathing feel more comfortable while sitting in bed—**acute LVF**.
2. Severe chest pain, anxious look, with hand on sternum **(Levine sign)**, sweating—**acute MI**.
3. Leaning forward with pain in the chest—**pericarditis**.
4. Pleurisy and dyspnoea—tend to lie on the diseased side.
5. Marked cachexia and wasting, **prominent eyeball seen in chronic CCF**, with low cardiac output.

Fundus Examination

In daily clinical practise, all doctors should know how to identify stages of hypertensive retinopathy in the fundus using an ophthalmoscope **as hypertension is the commonest disease in human being**.

Grade I	Increased light reflex with irregularity of retinal artery
Grade II	AV nipping, distention of vein
Grade III	Flame-shaped haemorrhage, cotton wool exudates, hard exudates
Grade IV	Papilloedema
Grades III and IV of hypertensive retinopathy	Seen in accelerated hypertension, which requires urgent medical treatment

Oral Examination

Petechiae in buccal mucosa: Infective endocarditis.
High-arched palate: Marfan's syndrome.
Large tongue:
   i. Amyloidosis
   ii. Restrictive cardiomyopathy
   iii. Myxoedema.

2

Dilated vein under the surface of tongue: Raised jugular venous pressure in chronic CCF with TR.

Eyes

- Mild jaundice, chronic congestive heart failure, pulmonary infarction.
- Ectopia lentis: Marfan's syndrome.
- Conjunctival petechiae: Infective endocarditis.

Corneal arcus: Around cornea white pigmentation as white rim, starts from the inferior part and then slowly encircles it, causings **premature IHD**.

Cyanosis

- It is due to low arterial oxygen saturation in blood (O^2 saturation below 92%).
- **Central:** Seen in under the surface of tongue, uvula and palatine mucosa.
- **Peripheral:** Tips of hands, feet, nose, more in cold climates.
- Central cyanosis, CHD (congenital heart disease) (cyanotic), Eisenmenger syndrome with R → L shunt, TOF, TGA, DORV with PS (pulmonary stenosis), TA (truncus arteriosus), tricuspid atresia.

Eisenmenger syndrome: Pulmonary hypertension in acyanotic CHD which later progresses to R → L shunt and cyanosis in **shunt lesions**. Develop earliest in VSD then in PDA, and after 30–40 years in ASD.

Oedema

- In CCF: Initially dependent oedema at feet and legs is noted and then progresses to ascites, in bedridden cases, oedema at sacral pad.
- The pressure at the bony joint should be applied for 1/2 minute, following which the depression persists for 1/2 minute.
- Rarely slight pitting oedema seen in obesity.
- Drug like NSAID can cause oedema.
- **Unilateral oedema:** Post-surgical harvesting of saphenous vein in CABG cases and in deep vein thrombosis.
- **Before oedema occurs, 2–3 kg weight increase is noted.**

Hands

Subungual splinter haemorrhages:

- Trauma
- Rarely infective endocarditis.

Proximal interphalangeal joint spindle-shaped, rheumatoid nodule on the extensor surface of the hand and forearm (in rheumatoid arthritis).

Nodules on proximal interphalangeal joints are seen in osteoarthritis.

Rheumatic arthritis does not affect hands, but large joints are affected. Few discrete nodules are seen on extensor surface of the elbow besides on the knuckle and suboccipital region—in **RHD** (rheumatic heart disease). In children arthralgia is seen more common than full-blown arthritis, in India.

- Holt-Oram syndrome—absence of thumb, ASD, common atrium
- Polydactyly, Eills Van Creveld syndrome

- Sweating of palms and tremors anxiety state.
- Transient malar cyanosis in very fair females—tight MS with low CO and pulmonary artery hypertension. Differential diagnosis, SLE.

Clubbing of Nails

- There is obliteration of angle at the base of the nail with skin—Grade I
- Clear clubbing with a soft nail bed and longitudinal curving of nail—Grade II
- Prominent drumstick appearance and gross clubbing—Grade III
- Clubbing with hypertrophic osteoarthropathy—Grade IV.

Causes

Cardiac: **Cyanotic congenital heart disease**, e.g. TOF (tetralogy of Fallot), TGA (transposition of great arteries) TAT (tricuspid atresia) TA (truncus arteriosus)

1. Infective endocarditis
2. Eisenmenger syndrome
3. Congenital (since birth): Both nails and toes affected
4. Noncardiac: Bronchogenic carcinoma, lung disease (lung abscess, bronchiectasis)
5. Ulcerative colitis.

Skin

- **Rheumatoid nodules** already mentioned.
- **Erythema marginatum:** Very rare in Indians. Only seen in very fair skinned people with rheumatic fever.
- Pigmentation (Brownish) seen after sun exposure, after long standing **amiodarone treatment**. It is very rare in Indian population, compared to the west.
- **Diagonal transverse earlobe crease—IHD**.

Arthritis

In children with rheumatic fever, arthritis is seen less commonly and mostly occurs as arthralgia. In **children, carditis is more common**. **More than 30% of patients may not give history of sore throat and arthritis**.

In adults with rheumatic fever get more active inflammation of joints compared to children. Rheumatic fever is still very common in Indian population. Its prevalence rate is **5–6 per 1000 population. Dramatic response to salicylate is a diagnostic clue**.

Rheumatoid arthritis shows classical proximal, interphalangeal joint spindle-shaped deformity, early morning stiffness and rarely, rheumatoid nodules may be seen.

Gouty arthritis, more suspected by history of acute painful, **metatarsophalangeal joint involvement**. Diuretic treatment may precipitate acute gout attack.

Fever in Case of Heart Disease

Normal body temperature is **37°C (98.6°F)**, with a variation of **36°–37.8°C. Fever is defined when temperature is more than 37.8°C, i.e. 100°F**. Fever in heart disease has a serious connotation. Short-term fever is due to viral and upper respiratory tract infection like in other people. But fever when it is of low grade and continuous, remittent and is lasting for **more than 2 weeks,** is **a serious clinical problem**.

In the presence of heart disease especially CHD/ valvular heart disease the following conditions should be looked for:

1. **Infective endocarditis**
2. **Pericarditis:** Rheumatic/tubercular/viral
3. **Rheumatic fever:** Relapse attack rather less common cause is to be excluded.
4. **Acute MI:** Fever seen in first **3rd to 7th day, low due to muscle necrosis**.

Infective endocarditis is a serious, treatable disease and should be suspected in any case of cardiac murmur, fever, splenomegaly and clubbing of nails. Arthralgia is seen in **40% of cases**. Skin lesion like Osler nodes and Janeway lesions are very rare in Indians. Rarely, fever may be absent in Infective Endocarditis when the patient is old and has congestive cardiac failure or renal failure. Instead of fever, the patient may have **sweating, weakness, malaise and arthralgia**.

If infective endocarditis is suspected patient is to be admitted immediately to the hospital and after aseptic precaution **10 cc blood drawn for blood culture and 5 cc each put in two blood culture bottles at earliest and sent immediately to hospital lab. There should be no delay in this job by nursing staff**.

If fever persists besides antibiotic treatment for infective endocarditis, then look for **IV site–phlebitis, IM—injection abscess**, drug fever.

Always exclude other common causes like malaria, tubereculosis, enteric fever, upper respiratory tract infection and urinary tract infection (UTI) and COVID-19—coronavirus in present era.

Fever with Polyarthritis

1. Rheumatic fever
2. Rheumatoid arthritis
3. SLE (systemic lupus erythematosus)
4. Reactive arthritis
5. UTI and enteric infection.

In rheumatic fever, a sequela to streptococcal throat infection, prompt response to aspirin is a good diagnostic point besides athralgia/flitting arthritis.

Fever in Case of IHD

1. Acute MI—low grade due to muscle necrosis, starts within 24–48 hours and may continue up to 7 days.
2. IV fluid and indwelling catheters in sick patient. Producing phlebitis most commonest cause.
3. Acute respiratory tract infection, UTI, may precipitate angina and aggravate CCF (congestive cardiac failure).

When infective endocarditis is suspected, look for the following common cardiac lesions:

1. Signs of MR (mitral regurgitation)
2. Signs of AR (aortic regurgitation)
3. Bicuspid aortic valve
4. VSD (ventricular septal defect)
5. Any prosthetic valve
6. PPM (permanent pace maker).

Chapter 3

Blood Pressure Evaluation

Blood pressure (BP) estimation is a very common procedure in daily clinical practice. Every patient must have his/her BP checked.

Physiologically BP is a lateral pressure exerted on the vessel wall by blood flow with each LV systole, determined by its stroke volume. The stroke volume × heart rate determines cardiac output (CO). Finally blood pressure is the product of CO and the peripheral vascular resistance. To summarise:

CO = Stroke volume × heart rate

BP = CO × peripheral vascular resistance

Normal BP in healthy adults is in between 110/70 and 130/80 mm.

BP estimation is the most important physical sign in the examination of the cardiovascular system. Hypertension is an important risk factor in **coronary heart disease, cerebrovascular and renovascular disease and diabetes mellitus**. If detected earlier its control can prevent and modify progress of these diseases.

Method of Measurement of BP

A Noninvasive/Indirect Method

Riva Rocci, an Italian physicist, discovered the **pneumatic cuff/manometer in 1896** and subsequent **discovery and use of arterial sounds by Korotkoff in 1905** established this technique as a standard method for measurement of blood pressure. In this method, an inflatable bladder is covered by non-distensible cuff is used to wrap arm/leg to occlude the artery. The bladder is connected to a **spring-mode aneroid meter**. It has replaced old Mercury manometer. It is **also connected to pressure bulb**. After the distal artery pulsation is occluded then gradually the pressure in the bladder is released at a rate of 2–3 mm/sec when Korotkoff sound is heard. The Korotkoff sound vary in intensity at different phases (Table 3.1).

The size of the bladder has been standardised for different sizes of arm/thigh at different ages. The width of the inflatable bladder should cover **40% of circumference**

Table 3.1: Phases of Korotkoff sound

Phase I	Onset of auditory sound–clear tapping sound. It is equivalent to systolic blood pressure
Phase II	Onset of swishing sound or murmur
Phase III	Loud murmur like sound
Phase IV	Sudden muffling of sound. It occurs 5–10 mmHg higher than true diastolic blood pressure
Phase V	Disappearance of sound = represents true diastolic blood pressure

at the mid-point of a limb on which it is used. Now circumference of limb is used as it can be measured easily. **On average adult a bladder of 12–14 cm width is used.** Length of the inflatable bladder should be twice the recommended width, i.e. **80% of circumference of limb used.**

The bladder should be applied directly over the compressive artery.

If too short bladder width is used, high recordings are noted and too large bladder will produce low readings.

The suggested sphygmomanometer cuff sizes in centimetre as per AHA (American Heart Association) recommendation is as follows (Table 3.2).

Table 3.2: Recommended cuff sizes as per AHA

Patient subset	*Arm circumference*	*Bladder width* (cm)	*Bladder length* (cm)
Child	13–20	8	13
Small adult	17–26	11	27
Standard adult	**24–32**	**13**	**24**
Large adult	32–42	17	32
Muscular and obese arm and thigh	45–50	20	42

Technique of Blood Pressure Estimation

1. Patient should have taken rest at least for 2 minutes in the physician's office and sitting on a chair is recommended to place an arm resting at heart level (Fig. 3.1).
2. **No caffeine used at least one hour before checking BP.**
3. **No smoking at least 15 minutes before BP estimation.**
4. Quite comfortable surroundings with friendly ambient temperature.
5. Proper size bladder with surrounding cuff should be wrapped around the arm and bladder should cover **at least two-thirds of length of the arm**. The lower **edge of cuff should be 2.5 cm above antecubital fossa.**

   The cuff should be of non-distensible material so that even pressure is exerted on extremity under cuff. Cuff can be of contact closure (Viceroy material), or bandage type. If cloth bandage type, cuff cover should be long enough to encircle arm several times with width extending beyond lower end of inflatable bladder (we in India still use these types).
6. The bladder should be inflated to occlude the brachial artery up to above 10 mmHg, the reading was taken by palpatory method for systolic BP.
7. Deflate gradually at a rate of 2–3 mmHg/sec.

The systolic pressure is noted at the appearance of the 1st Korotkoff sound and diastolic at disappearance of sound.

Two sets of readings should be taken at an **interval of two minutes.** If readings vary more than 5 mmHg additional reading should be taken.

In case of AR and children and hyperdynamic state, the diastolic BP is recorded when Korotkoff sounds are muffled because sound can be heard up to 0 mmHg. It should be recorded as 170/40+0 or 160/50+0. The Fig. 3.1 is showing correct method of blood pressure recording.

Normal variation: In normal persons mostly right and left arm pressures are equal, but right arm pressure may be higher by 10 mmHg than left arm.

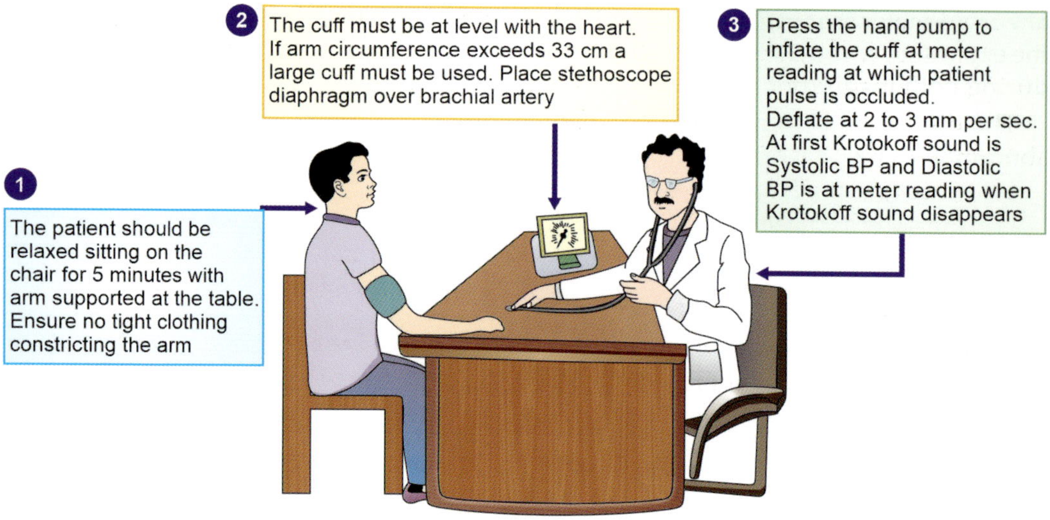

Fig. 3.1: Blood pressure measurement technique

Standing BP: If patient is more than 65 years, and in cases of hypertension on drug treatment, one must record standing BP after patient is standing for three minutes. Normally **systolic BP up to 20 mm fall and diastolic up to 10 mmHg can be noted**.

Common Causes of Unequal BP in Two Arms

1. Aortoarteritis (Takayasu syndrome)
2. Cardiogenic embolism of proximal brachial artery
3. Subclavian steal syndrome.

Blood Pressure Estimation in Lower Limb

It is specifically indicated in the following conditions:

1. Suspected aortoarteritis, coarctation of aorta
2. Peripheral arterial embolism
3. Unequal arterial pulsations any where
4. Grading of aortic regurgitation by Hill's sign if lower limb BP more than 20 mmHg compared to upper limb
   a. Grade I >20 mm 1 + AR
   b. Grade II >20–40 mm 2 + AR
   c. Grade III >40–60 mm 3 + AR
   d. Grade IV >60 mm 4 + AR

Other Clinical Signs Elicited by Aneuroid Meter

Pulsus paradoxus: Normally systolic BP falls during inspiration due to pooling of blood in pulmonary circulation and transient fall in LV filling volume. **Normally it falls by 8 mmHg. If it falls by more than this, it is abnormal and is called pulsus paradoxus.**

3

Using the sphygmomanometer patient is asked to breathe normally. Cuff is inflated above level of systolic pressure. Then deflate very slowly by 2–3 mmHg/sec. An aneuroid meter reading at which Korotkoff sound is heard intermittently is noted. It is the expiratory level. By further deflation, the Korotkoff sounds are continuously audible during both inspiration and expiration. That level is also recorded.

The difference between the two is noted as pulsus paradoxus more than 8 mm is abnormal.

When to look for pulsus paradoxus:

1. All cases of CCF without S_3 audible
2. Unexplained heart failure
3. Constrictive pericarditis.
4. Suspected cardiac tamponade (sudden increase in volume of pericardial fluid)
5. An acute episode of bronchial asthma.

Normally Pulsus Paradoxus is seen in:

- Pregnancy
- Exaggerated voluntary inspiration (student paradoxus)
- Extreme obesity.

Blood Pressure Alternans

Alternate strong and weak LV contraction produces pulse waves felt as weak and strong alternately. It is a sign of LV dysfunction. It is seen in cases of:

1. Aortic stenosis
2. Dilated cardiomyopathy
3. Severe AR.

Severe alternans may not be felt on pulse but can be appreciated by BP estimation. When Korotkoff sound alternates in intensity and changes in meter reading by >20 mmHg, it is significant.

Other uses of Aneroid

1. As venous tourniquet: To reduce venous return by applying on both thighs and arms and inflated up to below diastolic BP. Kept for 15 minutes and released and then rotated on all four limbs (an outdated procedure).
   - Used in acute pulmonary oedema
   - **To reduce AR by increasing PVR**.
2. In diagnosing: **Thrombocytopenia (Hess test)**. The cuff is tied around the arm and inflated midway between systolic and diastolic and kept for 5 minutes. Number of petechiae appearing in an area of 2.5 sqm on inner side of arm is noted. **Normally up to 20 are noted**. More than that is abnormal.
3. **Chvostek sign:** Carpopedal spasm on inflating cuff around post-tibial artery in cases of **hypocalcaemia**.

Ambulatory BP Measurement

Now commercially a large variety of reliable BP monitors are available which record BP continuously. They are based on heart stroke volume, and by electronic modification, a modified form of pulse wave is detected by a sensor placed on the brachial artery.

These monitors are programmed to record BP every 15–30 minutes throughout day and night while the patient goes about daily activities and during sleep. The readings are linked to a computer and histographic display of BP reading in relation to activity is available. Normal BP by ambulatory BP is lower than clinic reading mostly less than **135/85 mmHg** if BP is less than 10–20% during sleep. It is indicated to correctly evaluate hypertension drug treatment of patient and to avoid gross hypotension.

Indications of Ambulatory BP Monitoring

1. Where persistent clinic BP is higher to establish diagnosis of hypertension.
2. To exclude "White coat hypertension", i.e. high BP in doctor's office but normal at home.
3. To diagnose drug resistance and avoid drug-induced hypotension.
4. To evaluate autonomic dysfunction.

Self-Home Measurement of BP

With the availability of portable, electronic BP monitors, most patients will like to periodically check BP at home. The advantages are:

1. Excluding white coat hypertension.
2. Response to drug treatment.
3. Checking and encouraging patient's active compliance to treatment. Reduces cost of treatment.

Home BP above 135/80 is considered abnormal. All these instruments should be monthly validated and the reading checked with a standard aneroid meter.

Pseudohypertension

In elderly patients, rigid and calcified arteries may not easily collapse by pneumatic pressure in bladder of BP cuff and pulse felt after Korotkoff sound disappears. This gives a false high recording of systolic BP.

It is suspected when in an elderly patient without any target organ damage and any hypertensive retinopathic changes BP recording is high.

By Osler's test pseudohypertension can be excluded. The Osler's manoeuvre means that radial pulse continues to be palpable after the brachial artery gets occluded as an evidence of disappearance of Korotkoff sound.

Ankle–Brachial Index

This is a ratio of ankle BP to brachial BP. Normally, ankle BP is higher than brachial BP so the ratio is more than 1. The technique of recording ankle blood pressure by Doppler is shown in Fig 3.2, the position of the cuff, the Dorsalis pedis artery and Posterior Tibial artery are explained also.

Measure the upper limb systolic BP over brachial artery and ankle BP over posterior tibial artery ideally using. Doppler method or at least with usual aneroid meter with the cuff over the leg. Calculate the ratio of ankle-systolic BP to brachial. In peripheral vascular disease especially in diabetes this ratio is less than 1. A ratio of less than **0.7** indicates severe peripheral vascular disease due to atherosclerosis. In addition

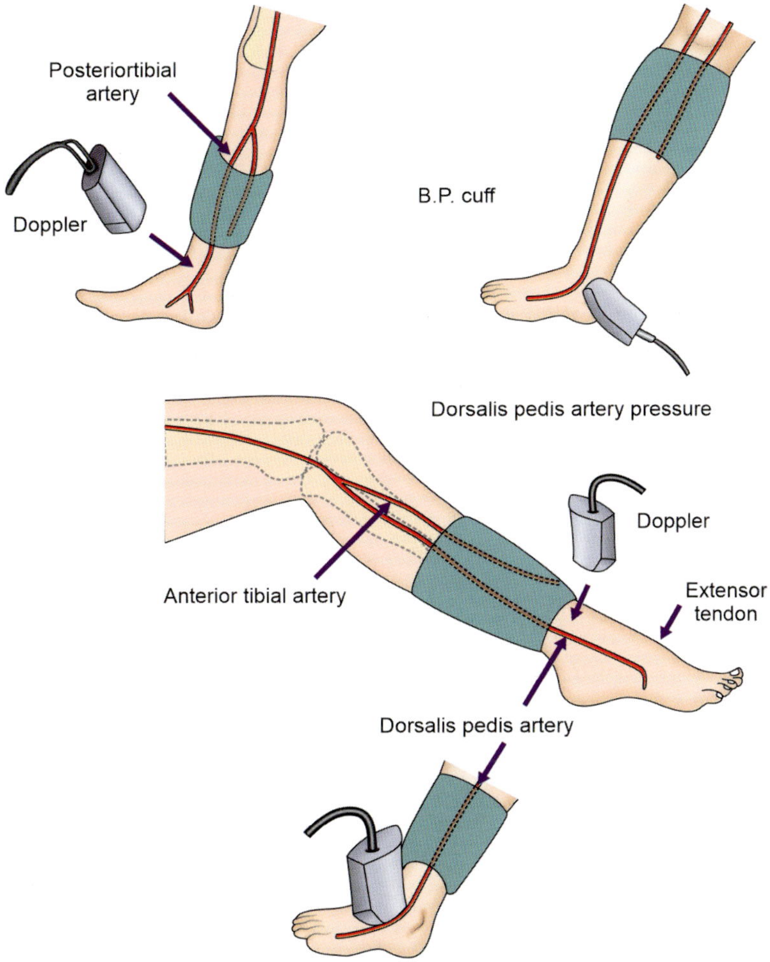

Fig. 3.2: Ankle systolic blood pressure evaluation

to its association with peripheral vascular disease, it is an important indicator of co-existing coronary heart disease as has been documented in recent prospective studies.

Chapter 4

Examination of Heart

Heart is an important single organ located in thorax in between two lungs. It supplies oxygenated blood from LV chamber via aorta and its branches (arteries) to all human body. The deoxygenated blood comes back to right side atrium via SVC and IVC → RA. From RA deoxygenated blood enters RV through tricuspid valve. RV pumps this blood to both the lungs via pulmonary arteries → capillaries in lungs where it gets oxygenated blood by breathing fresh air. This oxygenated blood returns to LV via pulmonary veins to LA to LV and then to aorta.

In clinical examination of heart, one should be very careful in examining the heart, the vital organ of human body. The doctor should follow the proper procedure as given in details in the next pages of this chapter. One should not miss any findings in a diseased heart. The clinician should correlate the findings of physical examination along with symptoms and with the help of ECG data he/she can come to correct diagnosis in most of the cases.

INSPECTION

Whole of anterior chest wall is bared of clothes and carefully inspected. When a lady patient (between 8 years and 80 years.) is examined a lady attendant (lady helper/staff nurse) or patient's father or mother, husband or sister must be present at the bed side. It is mandatory particularly when a male doctor is examining the female patient. In wards a good screen is used to cover all sides of patient's bed. Patient is asked to take deep breath, any limitation of chest wall movement noticed. Patient is asked to cough, any buldge in chest wall or parasternal area noted, e.g. aortic aneurysm can produce a visible buldge.

Note any systolic pulsation in precordium or any retraction at LV apex. Note the site of cardiac apex and any other abnormality. Any pulsation in suprasternal region, e.g. by aortic arch aneurysm or any prominent pulsation in neck vessel is noted. In epigastrium pulsation transmitted from the heart after post or inferior wall MI are noted. Notice any chest wall deformity or thoracic spine deformity like kyphosis or kyphoscoliosis.

Examiner while standing on foot side of patient, in a good light, can see minute cardiac pulsations very clearly, which may not be felt on pulsation, especially related to S4 heart sound. Hence, a good inspection can give us valuable data.

PALPATION

Clinical Importance of Apex Beat

Apex beat is outermost and lowermost point of cardiac pulsation in precordium, where finger is distinctly lifted. Normally it is located in 4th or 5th IC space inside mid-clavicular line and total area is covered by one finger (area of old 25 paisa coin).

Location: Normal apex is formed by LV. In palpating apex beat if one cannot locate apex in supine posture, turn the patient to left lateral position, apex beat can be easily felt and its quality can be made out.

The Location of Apex can Change due to Extracardiac cause

Shift to left: Fibrosis of the left lung, collapse of left lung or pneumothorax or pleural effusion on the right side.

Shift to right: Fibrosis of the right lung or collapse of right lung, pleural effusion on the left side.

Cardiac Abnormalities Detected at Apex Beat Examination/Types of Apex Beat

1. **Tapping apex:** Cardiac impulse is sudden and felt for very short time, i.e. 1/2 of systole seen in **mitral stenosis, in anxiety state and any event causing tachycardia. Tapping apex is due to palpable 1st heart sound**.
2. **Thrusting apex:** A vigorous non-sustained apex felt over wide area. Felt during whole of systole, is seen in volume loaded LV, e.g. AR, MR, VSD, cases with large shunt.
3. **Heaving apex or sustained apex:** Vigorous and sustained apex, rises slowly and occupies whole of systole, seen in aortic stenosis and hypertension.

   Systole is the time interval between first heart sound and second heart sound, diastole is time interval between second heart sound and first heart sound. These fundamental cardiac events have been taught during the MBBS course in physiology and clinical medicine.

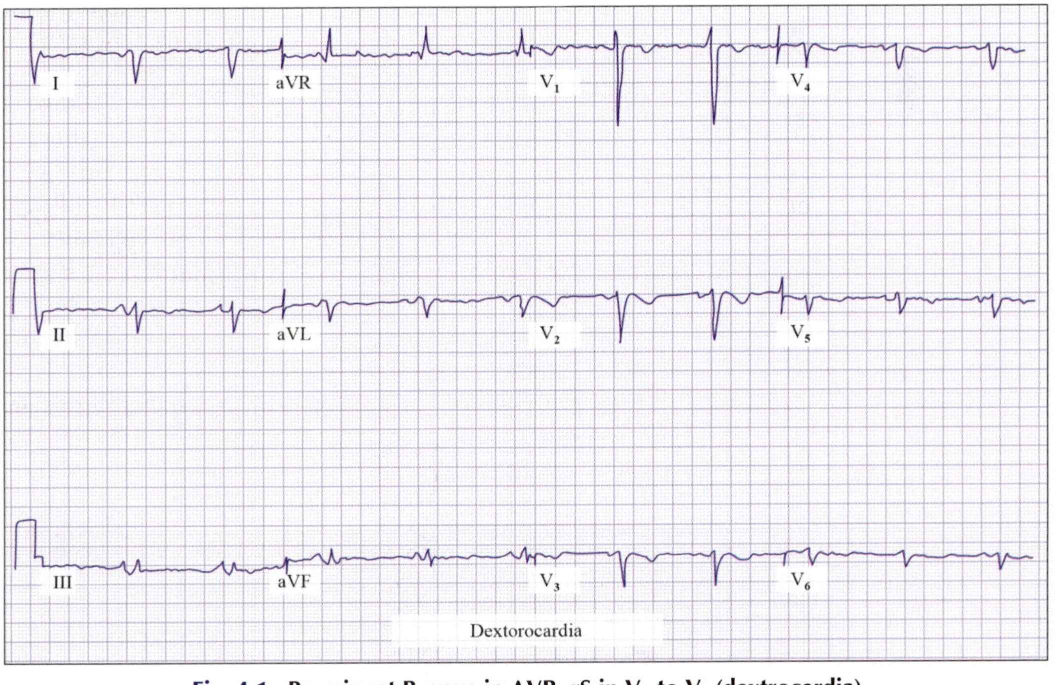

Fig. 4.1: Prominent R wave in AVR, rS in V_1 to V_5 (dextrocardia)

4. **Double apex:** Two pulsations felt with each cardiac contraction, it is due to palpable atrial impulse in HOCM and in ventricular aneurysm (due to a outward movement in systole).
5. **Right ventricular apex:** When RVH is severe, the apical pulsation is not felt at usual site but a systolic pulsation is felt in LPS area and a negative pulsation at apex site. Cardiac pulsation is felt in epigastrium just below the ribs mostly in this right ventricular pathology.
6. **Impalpable apex:** Normally in obesity and in diseases like emphysema, pericardial effusion, left side pleural effusion apex cannot be felt.
7. In rare cases the heart is situated in right hemithorax, i.e. dextrocardia. Sometimes the whole body viscera usually on the left side is embryologically changes to right side. Liver on the left side, stomach on right side in dextrocardia. ECG shows prominent R wave in V_1, V_3r, V_4r, and rS wave in V_1 to V_5 (Fig. 4.1).

JUGULAR VENOUS PULSE (JVP)

JVP term means Jugular venous pulsation of right internal jugular vein. These venous waves are seen coming through superior vena cava from right atrium, with which it is in direct communication. So in cardiac contraction and relaxation, whatever pressure changes take place in the cardiac chambers these are transmitted directly to **right internal jugular vein**. Patient reclines at 45° in bed for examination of JVP pulsation in right internal jugular vein. **Jugular vein pulsation** is not commonly seen since it has valves and it passes through scalenus neck muscle which can obstruct the waves. **External jugular vein can be used if pulsation is visible in it. For JVP examination right side of neck is examined**.

In neck: We examine JVP watching right internal jugular pulsation on right side of neck which are seen more **prominent as descent waves**. These pulsations are seen with all beats. Best seen just above clavicle, between two head of scalenus muscle. If we put pressure at root of neck (above clavicle) pulsations disappear.

Normally in JVP three waveforms are seen as ascent waves and two descent waves, **especially descent waves** are more prominent (Fig. 4.2).

A wave is seen as upward pulsation before carotid pulse produced by right carotid artery pushing right jugular vein upwards pulsation before the carotid artery, pulse. This A wave is also due to SVC filling of right atrium occur (Fig. 4.3).

C wave is due to upward movement of TV (tricuspid valve) in right atrium during atrial systole A and C waves are usually seen together.

X descent is seen due to pulling down of right AV ring of tricuspid valve at the start of right ventricle systole. V ascent wave is due to filling of right ventricle from right atrium.

Y descent filling of right ventricle at beginning of diastole of RV. VY descent is seen in the venous filling of RV.

Measurement: Patient sitting in bed with back support at 45° and we note the upper level of internal jugular vein pulsation. Keep a 6″ ruler in horizontal plane at this level. Then keep another ruler scale at sternal angle level. With third ruler measure the vertical height of JVP pressure between the two horizontal rulers. Normal is 0–4 cm measured by 3rd ruler kept vertically. Right atrial pressure is +5 cm + JVP as measured (Fig. 4.4).

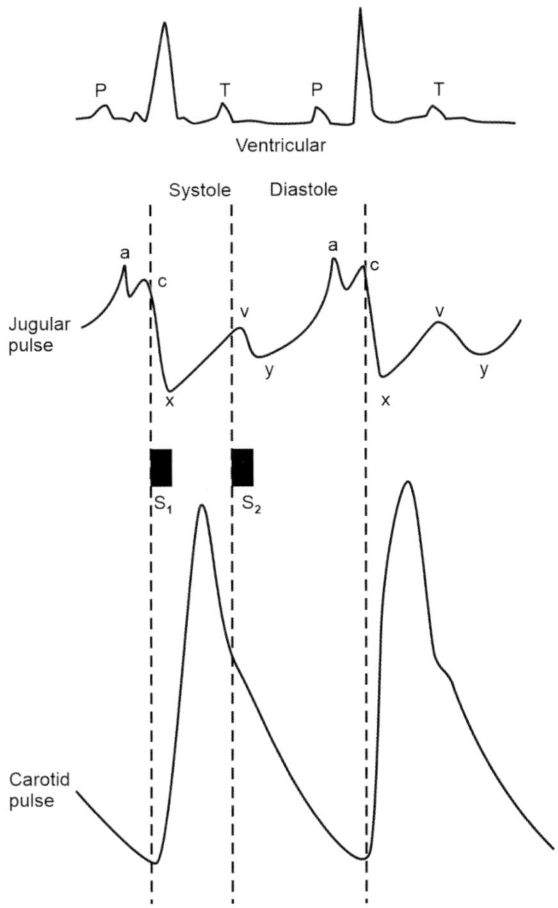

Fig. 4.2: ECG, JVP, heart sounds and carotid pulse wave correlation in normal person

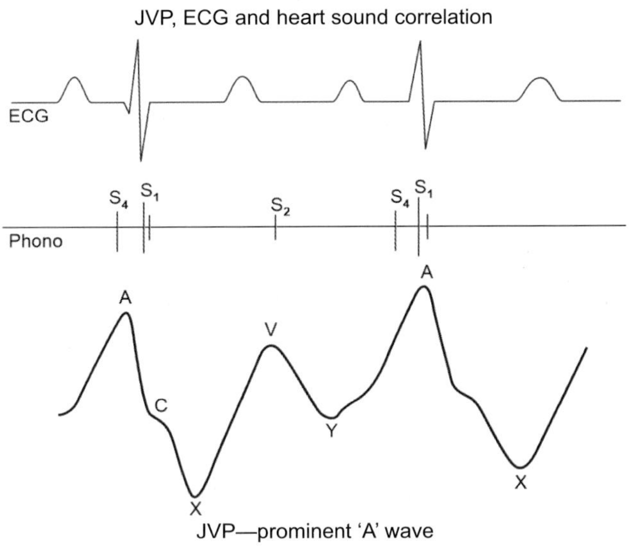

Fig. 4.3: Prominent 'A' wave in JVP seen in pulmonary stenosis, tricuspid atresia, RVH

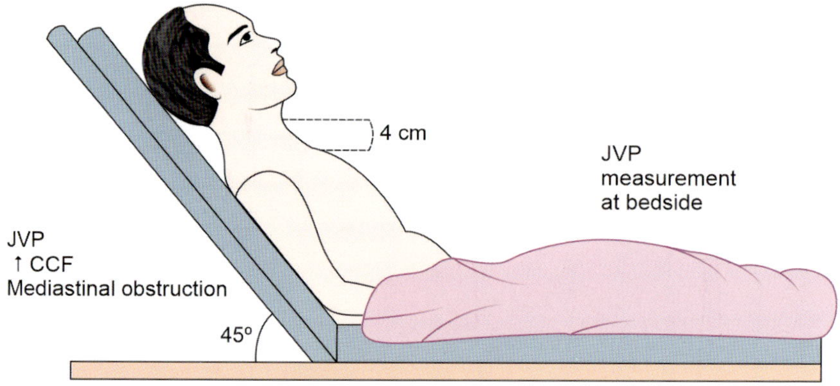

Fig. 4.4: **Method: Three 6″ scales required. Two such scales are placed horizontally at the upper level of JVP pulsation and at sternal angle level with 3rd vertical scales distance is measured between horizontal scales, it is JVP in cm**

Causes of Raised JVP

1. Congestive cardiac failure.
2. Superior vena cava obstruction, e.g. by constrictive pericarditis.
3. Mediastinal tumours (superior vena cave obstruction) non-pulsatile waves.
4. Over transfusion of IV fluids (commonest cause).

Prominent A Wave Seen in

- Pulmonary stenosis.
- RVH (right ventricular hypertrophy).
- Tricuspid atresia.
- Irregulary large A wave called **cannon waves** are seen in complete AV block since right atrium contracts on closed right AV valve (Fig. 4.5).
- Regular **cannon** waves are seen in junctional rhythm.
- **A wave absent in AF**.
- **Large V wave** seen in tricuspid regurgitation.
- Rapid V/Y descent seen with CCF and in cardiac tamponade (Fig. 4.6).

ARTERIAL PULSE

It is an important sign of arterial circulation and is felt as a positive pulsation at peripheral arteries with each heart beat (LV contraction).

The commonly examined **radial pulse. Radial artery pulse is felt at lower end of radius bone**. It tells us about rate, and rhythm of heart while with carotid pulse, amplitude and waveforms are analysed.

Normally, examiner should feel both radials, brachials, carotids, femorals and dorsalis pedis artery to find out any discrepancy and to detect distal arterial block. Each carotid artery in neck is felt separately.

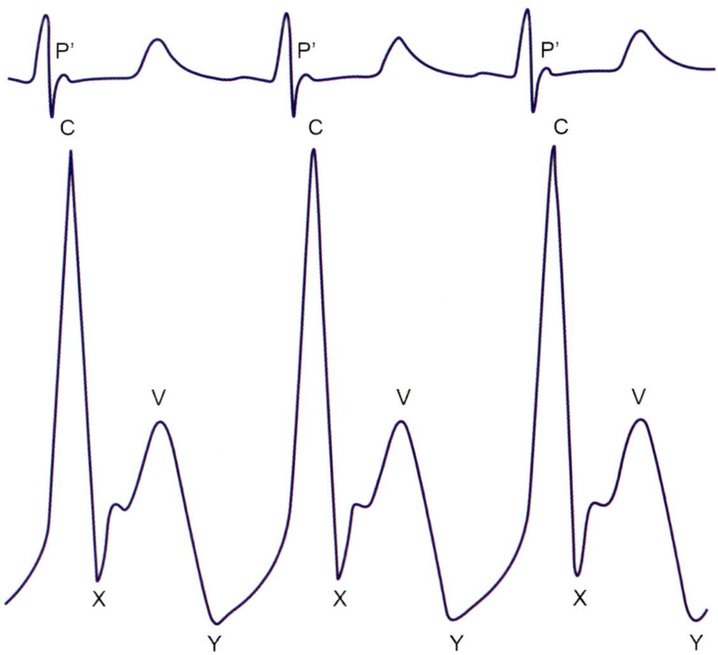

JVP and ECG correlation, cannon waves "C"
Regular cannon waves (C) are seen with junctional rhythm with 1:1 retrograde atrial activation (p')

Fig. 4.5: JVP—regular cannon 'C' wave

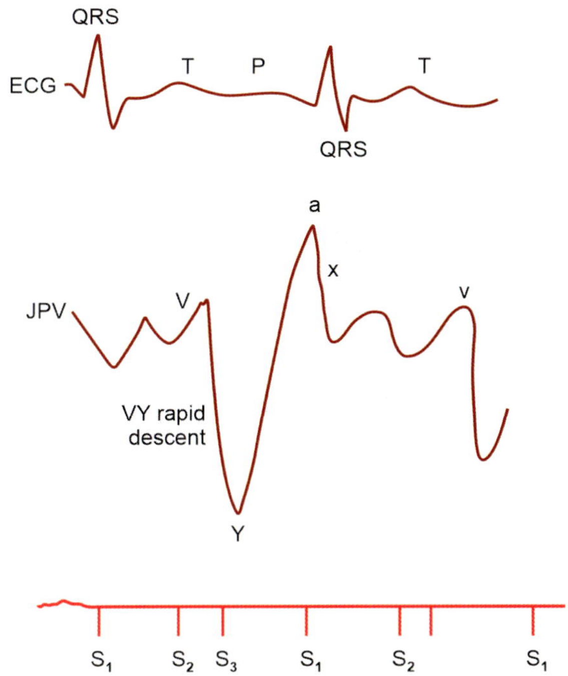

Fig. 4.6: JVP, ECG, heart sound correlation in case of cardiac temponade

Medical students must have wrist watch and not time the arterial pulse with the mobile (**please grown up medico girls and boys**. Note my advice).

Rate

Normal: 60 to 100 beats per minute. If rate more than 100 (tachycardia) seen in **fever, exercise, anxiety state. Thyrotoxicosis and cardiac failure and haemorrhage any where** and on drugs like salbutamol and beta agonists drugs. If rate is <60 per minute, it is called **sinus bradycardia**.

Causes

1. Trained athlete
2. Raised intracranial pressure
3. Complete AV block
4. Sick sinus disease
5. Obstructive jaundice
6. Drug effects, e.g. beta blocker
7. Hypothyroidism, hypothermia and vasovagal syncope.

Rhythm: Each pulse beat is separated from the preceding one and that following it by regular interval.

Normally heart rate during inspiration increases and in expiration decreases, it is called sinus arrhythmia.

Sinus arrhythmia is regularly irregular pulse: One feels dropping of pulses.

1. Incomplete heart block also causes regularly irregular pulse.

Irregularly irregular pulse:

The interval in between each beat is different and it changes with the beats. Most important cause is:

Atrial fibrillation: In this the pulse rate is less than heart rate counted by stethoscope at cardiac apex. This is called pulse deficit (>10).

To confirm atrial fibrillation auscultation of heart is superior method.

Multiple multifocal VPC cause irregular pulse but after exercise it tends to disappear. Best conformation is by ECG examination which shows varying RR interval, i.e. distance between 2 RR waves of ECG is always different.

Amplitude: It is judged by movement of palpating finger on arrival of pulse wave.

Large amplitude or large volume pulse is caused (Fig. 4.7):

a. Leakage of blood from AO into LV.
   Aortic regurgitation PDA, AV fistula.
   A pulse with brisk rise and fall is called **Water Hammer pulse** elicited by lifting and holding of arm it with grip of hand above the heart level.
b. Increased flow through dilated arteries: Thyrotoxicosis, pregnancy, anaemia.
c. Increased LV stroke volume–severe bradycardia.
d. In old people with loss of arterial elasticity, a normal pulse volume produces large pulse amplitude seen in carotids.

Low amplitude: Due to reduced stroke volume, e.g. shock, sinus tachycardia, LV failure, mitral stenosis, aortic stenosis.

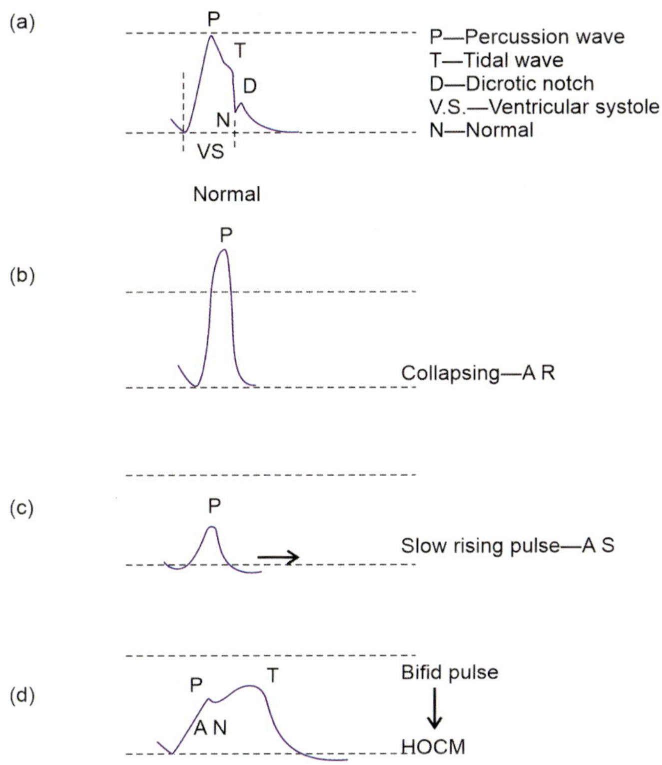

Fig. 4.7: Common types of arterial pulses

In aortic stenosis we get a slow rising pulse called **anacrotic pulse** specially seen at carotid pulse. In relation of amplitude we feel two pulse beats in each systole.

It is seen in:

1. HOCM (hypertrophic obstructive cardiomyopathy) called pulsus bisferiens.
2. Aortic stenosis and regurgitation.

In certain cases the amplitude of femoral pulse is much delayed compared to radial or carotid called **radiofemoral delay** seen in **coarctation of aorta and aortoarteritis (Takayasu syndrome)**.

In old age carotid artery pulsation may be diminished or absent in atherosclerosis. When we can listen a bruit over carotid it may be cause of CV accident in patient of hemiplegia.

In cases of AF with MVD or infective endocarditis peripheral arterial emboli occur and corresponding pulse will be absent.

TYPES OF ARTERIAL PULSE PATTERN

1. **Pulsus alternans:** Rate is regular but one pulse beat is with large amplitude and other is of small amplitude, e.g. in LV failure.
2. **Pulsus paradoxus:** It is an exaggeration of normal phenomenon. Normally during inspiration blood pressure (systolic) falls by 8 mmHg, since inspiratory pooling of blood in lungs, reduces LV venous return and hence reduced LV stroke volume and fall in BP.

If this phenomenon is exaggerated then we call it pulsus paradoxicus. Here the pulse disappears at wrist but heart sounds are audible.

Causes

1. Cardiac tamponade/constrictive pericarditis.
2. Restrictive cardiomyopathy in these diseases, there is decrease in diastolic filling volume of heart by tense fluid in pericardial sac or rigid pericardium. Here on inspiration, the increase in the space is not available for filling of LV ventricle. Hence, reduction in CO and decreased blood pressure.
3. In bronchial asthma and COPD the powerful inspiratory effort to increase inspiratory capacity further reduces the flow of blood to heart, hence reduced LV, CO and BP.

Method of Detection of Pulsus Paradoxus

Normally in inspiration BP falls by 8 mmHg.

Patient is sitting comfortably on the chair. Aneroid meter tied to the arm, and patient is asked to breathe normally. Cuff is inflated above systolic BP level, and then deflated very slowly by 2–3 mm/per sec. The level at which Korotkoff sounds are heard intermittently. It is expiratory level. By further deflation Korotkoff sounds are continually heard both during inspiration and expiration, this level is recorded the difference two levels is pulsus paradoxicus. Normally not more than 10 mmHg.

Change in the Pulse Wave Format

The pulse wave form is best appreciated in carotid pulse.

Normally, in pulse wave felt at carotid there is initial peak and rapid ascent occurs in 1st half of systole and no wave felt at ascending limb. As the patient gets older. The peak is rounded is delayed but rise is sharp. A very sharp pulse with rapid rise and fall occurs in *water hammer pulse*. This type of pulse is seen in AR, PDA and AV fistulae.

Pulsus bisferiens: It is term used when one feels extra beat (VPC) alternately with normal pulse. After VPC there is compensatory pause. There is alteration occurring regularly in pulse. Here weak beat follows the short interval and strong beat long interval. It is seen in HOCM (Fig. 4.8).

Percussion

In examination of heart. It is not of much value except in cases of moderate or severe pericardial effusion. Outer cardiac border are located beyond normal site. It is especially noted in 3rd or 4th intercostal spaces by percussion dullness on both right and left borders of heart.

Auscultation

Stethoscope with both chest and bell pieces is used for auscultation. Systematically all areas of precordium are auscultated as shown in Fig. 4.9. These areas are shown on the next page.

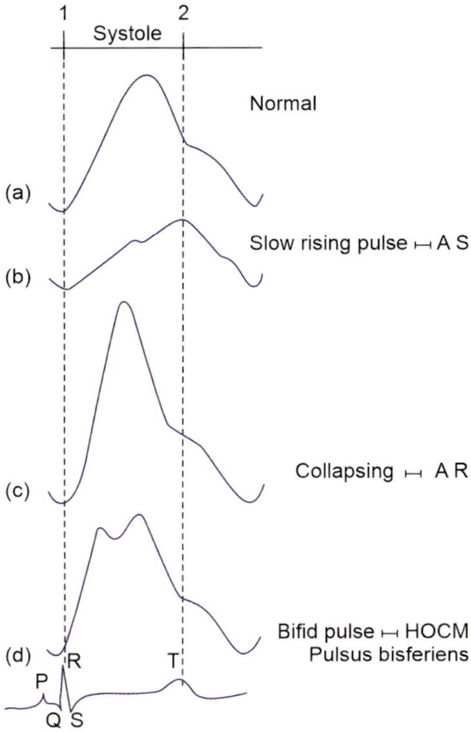

Fig. 4.8: Arterial pulses: Normal and abnormal

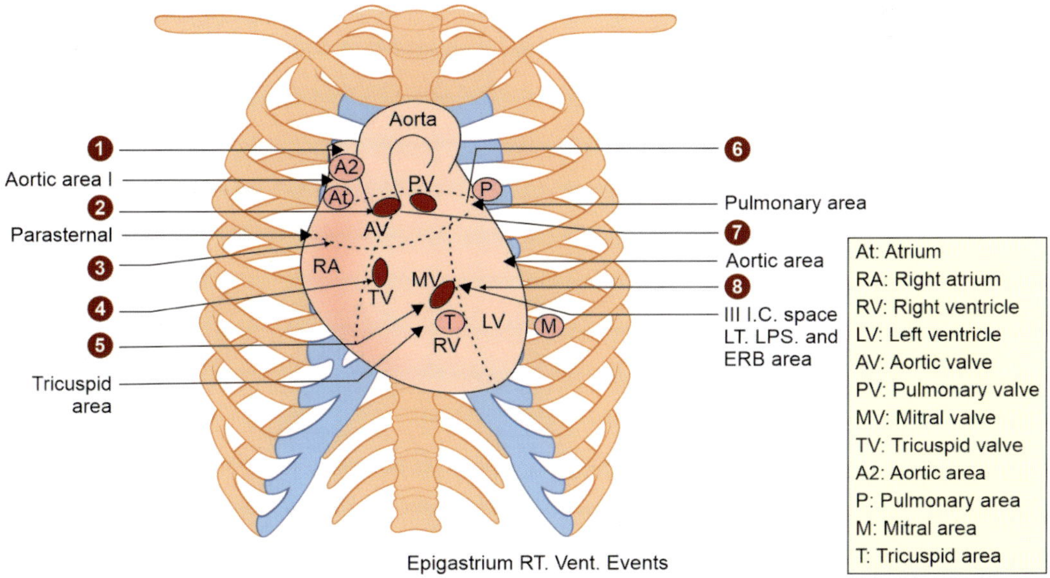

Fig. 4.9: Chest wall: Auscultatory areas of heart over cardiac valves

(1) Superior vena cava, (2) aortic valve, (3) base of the heart, (4) tricuspid valve, (5) mitral valve, (6) left atrial appendage, (7) pulmonary valve, (8) pulmonary artery.

Heart Sounds

Heart sounds are heard over precordium with stethoscope. With the help of stethoscope two heart sounds are heard normally. In younger age group 3rd heart sound is sometimes heard in younger athletes and young ladies.

First heart sound (S_1) is produced by closure of mitral valve and to some extent by Tricuspid valve. Best heard by chest piece and it is low pitched compared to 2nd heart sound which is high pitched. S_1 is best heard at apex (Fig. 4.10).

Second heart sound (S_2) is produced by closure of aortic and pulmonary valves, S_2 is usually use a single sound, heard at the apex.

In pulmonary area both components of S_2 (A_2 and P_2) are heard normally. Especially in inspiration (Fig. 4.11).

Physiologically S_2 is louder than S_1, especially in thin individual.

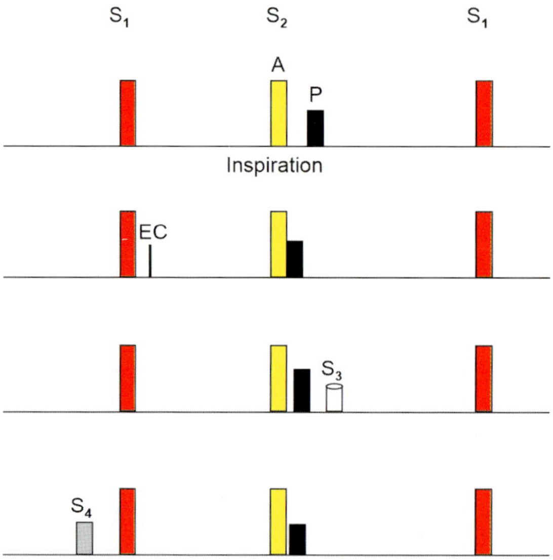

Heart Sounds

S_1–Produced by closure of mitral valve and 25% produced by closure of tricuspid valve best heard with chest piece at mitral area.

S_2–Closure of aortic valve (A_2) and closure of pulmonary valve (P_2).

S_3–Due to rapid ventricular filling when LV dilated and also MV ring dilated.

Soft dull sound in mid-diastole in LVF.

S_4–Diastolic sound at end of diastole in cases of LVH (HOCM) and IHD due to ↓ compliance of both ventricles, a high-pitched sound.

In inspiration A_2. P_2 wide as p_2 is delayed by large RV end-diastolic volume following blood pooling in capillaries of lung during inspiration, A_2 occurs earliest as LV end-diastolic volume is less due less LA output to LV. **In expiration single A_2P_2.**

Fig. 4.10: Normal heart sounds

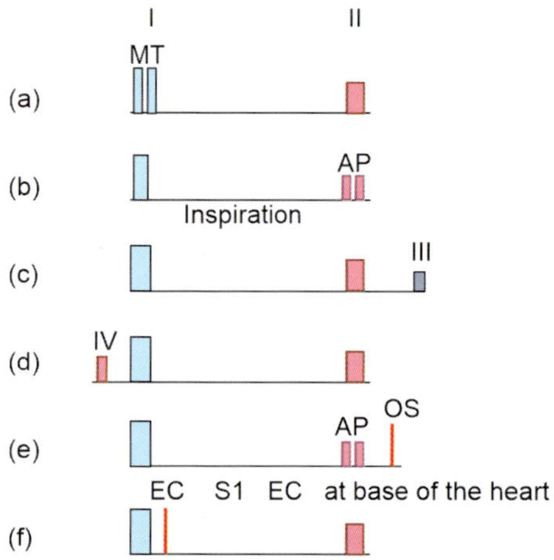

In Inspiration A_2. P_2 wide as p_2 is delayed by large pulmonary end-diastolic volume following blood pooling in capillaries in inspiration, A_2 occurs earliest as LV end-diastolic volume is less due less LA output to LV.

(a) Splitting of first heart sound/mitral and tricuspid components
(b) Splitting of S_2 (A_2P_2)
(c) III heart sound
(d) IV heart sound, single S_2
(e) Splitting of S_2 (A_2–P_2) with OS

OS is opening snap a loud high-pitched sound heard in diastole at mitral area. When present it indicates MV fit for mitral balloon valvuloplasty

Fig. 4.11: Normal and abnormal heart sounds with respiratory variations

4

Pathologically–Louder S_1

1. Mitral stenosis
2. Thyrotoxicosis
3. Any disease where there is short P–R interval in ECG like WPW syndrome.

Muffled or Absent Heart Sound in:

1. Obesity and emphysema.
2. Mitral regurgitation.
3. Calcific mitral stenosis.
4. Impaired LV function, e.g. in MI (myocardial infarct cases) S_1 is best heard at mitral area and it sounds as "Luv".

Second heart sound: It sounds as "Dub". It is produced by closure of aortic and pulmonary valve. Best heard at pulmonary and aortic area. It is high-pitched sound heard with diaphragm of stethoscope. 2nd heart sound has two components: Aortic closure (A_2) and pulmonary closure (P_2), is heard best in pulmonary area. At apex only A_2 is heard (Fig. 4.12).

In expirations: Both are heard as single component in pulmonary area.

In inspirations: A_2 and P_2 both components of S_2 are heard separately, due to increase in right ventricular filling volume taking prolonged time. Hence, P_2 closure is delayed. At the same time, more pooling of blood in pulmonary capillaries with inspiration causes decrease LV venous return and hence LV stroke volume is less and LV systole completes earlier and hence A_2 closure earlier.

In expiration: The process is reversed.

In inspiration: Normal splitting (in young children).

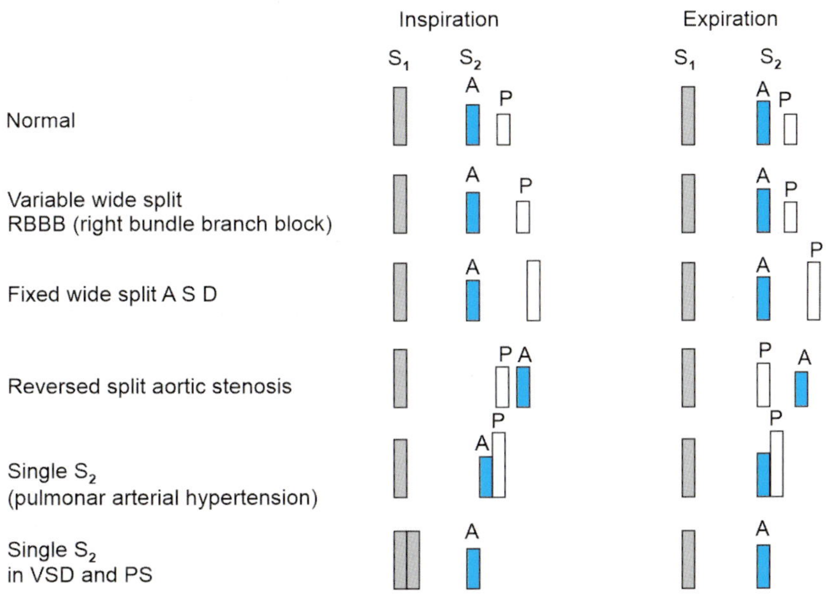

Fig. 4.12: Respiratory variations in heart sounds S_1 and S_2

Wide Physiological Splitting (Fig. 4.13)

In RBBB and pulmonary stenosis as RV systolic phase is prolonged hence P_2 is delayed.

Reversed Splitting

Here A_2 follows in P_2. It is seen in LVF, Aortic stenosis and LBBB, due to these diseases LV systole is prolonged, and hence A_2 comes after P_2.

Fixed Splitting and Wide (Fig. 4.13)

In ASD, there is shunting of blood from LA → RA. Hence whatever changes in RV and LV inflow volume occur in inspiration and expiration get nullified by shunt and there is some degree of RBBB and pressure in LA and RA are equal. Hence it causes **wide fixed split of A_2 P_2**. Other rare case of fixed split is anomalous pulmonary venous drainage.

S_2 (Intensity)

- Loud sound A_2 is **heard in hypertension**
- Soft/dull A_2: Aortic valvular stenosis, and CCF (low CO)
- **Loud P_2 is** heard in pulmonary arterial hypertension
- **Low intensity P_2**: Pulmonary stenosis valvular.

Third Heart Sound (S_3)

It is a low frequency sound best heard with bell of stethoscope after S_2 in diastolic phase. A soft **thudding noise**. It is due to rapid ventricular filling and can have LV or RV origin.

Site: Heard best in LPS 3rd intercostal space (ErB area) (RV) (Fig. 4.9) and at apex or at apex only (LV).

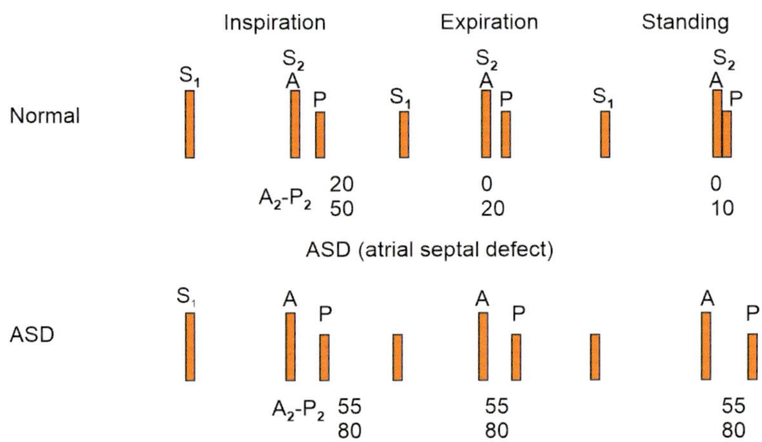

Inspiration: A_2-P_2 wide as P_2 is delayed by large pulmonary end-diastolic volume following of blood pooling in capillaries in inspiration, A_2 occurs earliest as LV end-diastolic volume is less due less LA output to LV.

In expiration single A_2P_2

Wide fixed split in ASD as LA → RA shunt equalizes both LV end-diastolic volume and RV end-diastolic volume.

Fig. 4.13: Respiratory variations in S_2 (A_2 P_2)

Causes

Physiological

In normal—healthy children, young adult, pregnancy, athletes.

Pathological

When LV is dilated and/or LV diastolic volume is increased there is rapid filling. It is seen in:

1. LV failure **(sound of cardiac disease)**
2. MR
3. Cardiomyopathies, e.g. postpartum cardiomyopathy.

When in heart failure 3rd heart sound is heard with tachycardia, the sound produce a cadence of galloping horse called LV Gallop.

Fourth Heart Sound (S_4)

It is also diastolic sound, produced by atrial contraction just before S_1. It is soft thud and is better **seen than felt at apex**.

Normally: In elderly people above 60 years.

Pathologically: When LV is hypertrophied or has lost compliance due to IHD, so to have more diastolic filling atrial contraction occurs to boost cardiac output.

Hence S_4 sound of **cardiac stress**

- LVH (hypertension)
- HOCM
- IHD.

Summation Gallop: With tachycardia diastole is shortened and with LVF in Advanced stage, both S_3 and S_4 are present. If heard simultaneously it is **Summation Gallop**, heard like a galloping horse.

The other abnormal sounds heard are:

1. **Ejection clicks:** High frequency sound heard best over pulmonary and aortic areas after S_1, best with diaphragm in case of valvular aortic stenosis (distance of S_1-EC is constant both in inspiration and expiration) click indicates valve is mobile and not calcified.
   Pulmonary stenosis: Valvular type mild and moderate EC is heard becomes less on inspiration and more on expiration. In inspiration more RV inflow causes premature opening of valve cusps.
2. **Mid-systolic clicks:** In MVP (mitral valve prolapse) due to sudden systolic tension on valve leaflet which prolapses in LV, on standing loud click is heard. It may or may not be accompanied by late systolic murmur.

Cardiac Murmurs

Cardiac murmurs are audible vibrations due to increased turbulence in the blood flow across the cardiac valves. They are classified as per their location in cardiac cycle. Systolic murmurs are heard in systolic phase between 1st heart sound (S_1) and 2nd heart sound (S_2–A^2P^2) and diastolic murmurs are heard in diastolic phase of cardiac cycle between S_2 and S_1.

Differential diagnosis of diastolic murmurs in apical region. The causes are (Fig. 4.14):

1. **Mitral stenosis:** It is most important cause. Here murmur is mid-diastolic and then continues up to pre-systole and then pre-systolic accentuation of murmur due to

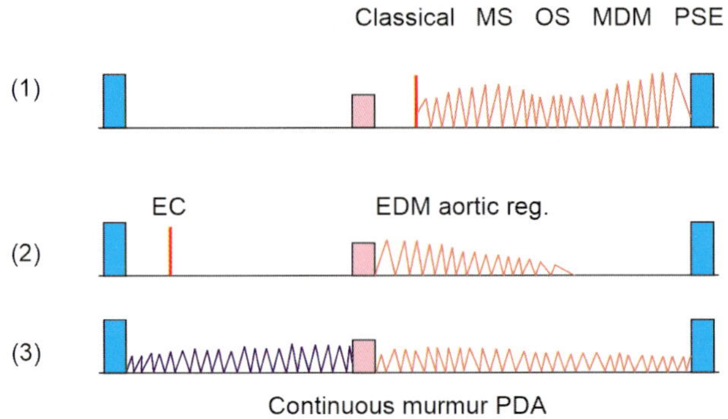

1. Typical auscultatory features in **mitral stenosis** (loud first heart sound, opening snap followed by mid-diastolic murmur (MDM) and presystolic murmur (PS).
2. Typical auscultatory finding in **aortic incompetence** (early decrescendo diastolic murmur) heard best over second aortic area and along sternal border.
3. Typical auscultatory findings in **patient of ductus arteriosus** (continuous murmur throughout systole and diastole).

Fig. 4.14: Common causes of diastolic murmurs

atrial contraction. When there is atrial fibrillation presystolic components are not heard. Murmur is rough rumbling, and best heard in left lateral sternal area more after exercise. Rheumatic heart disease is commonest cause of MS.

Longer the murmur severe the mitral stenosis (MS): In most cases it is preceded by **opening snap** which is **loud sound (OS)** means mitral valve is good for valvoplasty.

2. **Other conditions with increased flow of blood across the mitral valve:**
   i. VSD of L → R shunt
   ii. PDA of L → R shunt.
3. In some cases of excess mitral regurgitation, regurgitant volume from LA when flows back to LV short mid-diastolic murmur is produced.
4. In aortic regurgitation due to post-displacement of pressure over AML by regurgitation, diastolic murmur called **Austin Flint murmur** is produced.
5. In acute rheumatic fever AML is thickened its roughness produce relative MS, causing obstruction to blood flow to produce short MDM called **Carey Coomb murmur**. Heard in acute rheumatic carditis in rheumatic fever.
6. In LA myxoma: Diastolic murmur changes with posture of patient and is more on standing.
7. In constrictive pericarditis construction of MV ring from outside produces obstruction and can cause diastolic murmur. Rare cause.
8. Murmur of tricuspid stenosis may be heard at LPSE and mitral area and confused with MS but it increases on inspiration.

Benign or Innocent Cardiac Murmur

These are murmurs heard in precordium in the absence of any heart disease or disease of coronary circulation.

Causes: They are common in **children and young adults** and after age of 25 years in **hyperdynamic states like anaemia, pregnancy, hyperthyroidism and anxiety**. Chest deformity like straight back syndrome and funnel chest.

These murmurs are mostly short ejection systolic of grade I and grade II.

4

Site: Best heard over the pulmonary area which is also called **area of Auscultatory romance.** In school children these murmur are heard in 37% of boys and 51% of girls. Whenever there is doubt before we pronouce, judgement on significance of such murmur, patient should be referred to a cardiologist, who may do echocardiography to finally decide the cause of murmur.

Venous Hum: A continuous murmur heard in children by placing stethoscope just above sternal end of clavicle, obliterated by compression of internal jugular vein.

Causes and Differential Diagnosis of Systolic Murmur Over Mitral Area (Fig. 4.15)

The **organic** systolic murmurs over mitral area are mostly pansystolic start with S_1 and mostly extending right upto S_2.

The Most Common Causes are:

1. **Mitral regurgitation:** In our country RHD is still common cause below 40 years. The pansystolic murmurs is conducted to axilla and even up to thoracic spine and with the soft MDMs (mid-diastolic murmur) heard. So auscultate right up to spine. A_2P_2 may show wide split in inspiration as LV systole prolongs and A_2 is delayed (Fig. 4.16).
2. **IHD and MI:** Due to papillary muscle dysfunction poor compliance of mitral valve produces MR. The murmur is mostly pansystolic but may be mid-systolic with delayed onset. It had characteristic cooing character and heard best at edge of LPS area (Erb area) 3rd IC space.
3. **Mitral valve prolapse:** Mid/late systolic murmur occurs following a click more on standing murmurs becomes more prominent. Any manoeuvres which reduces LV. Volume increases intensity of murmur.

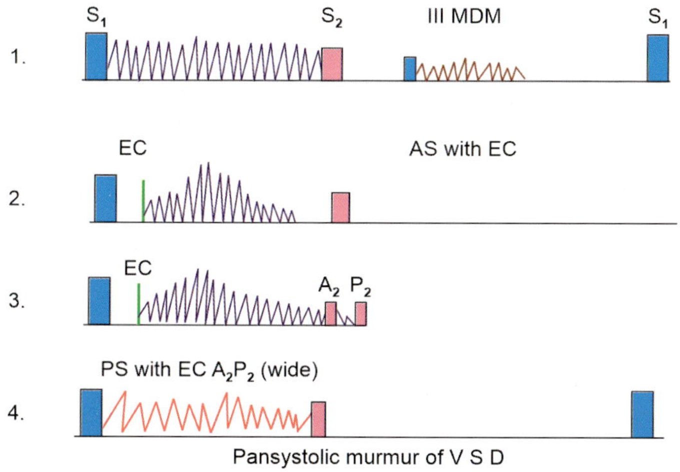

1. Typical auscultatory features in **organic mitral incompetence** (pansystolic murmur, third heart sound followed by mid-diastolic flow murmur).
2. Typical auscultatory signs in **aortic stenosis** (ejection click followed by mid-systolic murmur) heard over aortic area.
3. Typical auscultatory signs in **pulmonary stenosis** [ejection click (EC) followed by crescendo–decrescendo murmur with wide splitting of second heart sound] heard over pulmonary areas.
4. Pansystolic murmur of VSD heard left 4th intercostal space LPSE.

Fig. 4.15: Common systolic murmurs

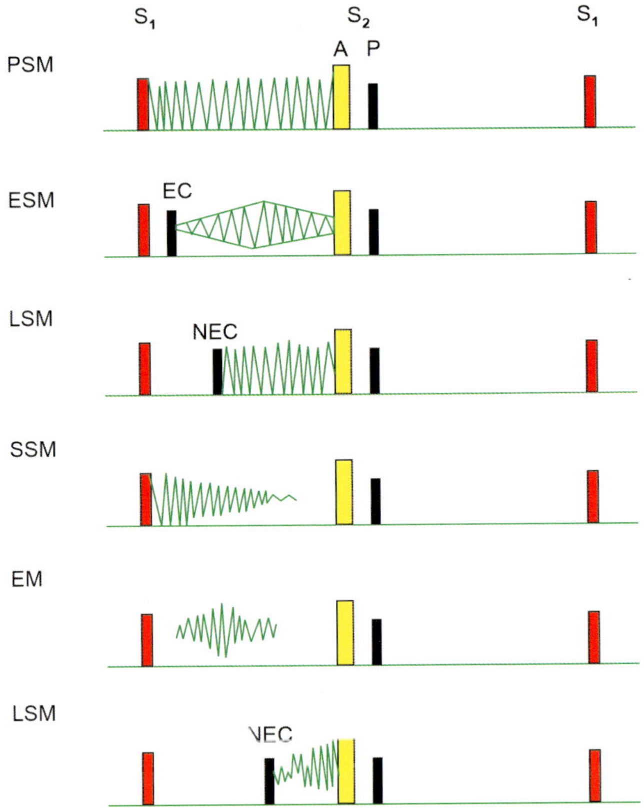

Definitions of systolic murmurs:

PSM Pansystolic murmur starts with first heart sound and ends with second heart sound of that side (A_2 or P_2).

ESM Ejection systolic murmur starts after first heart sound and ends with or before second heart sound of that side.

LSM Late systolic murmur starts well after first heart sound and ends with second heart sound of that side.

SSM Short systolic murmur may start with or after first heart sound and ends well before second heart sound.

EM Ejection murmur starts after first heart sound and ends well before second heart sound.

Fig. 4.16: Systolic murmurs

4. **Tricuspid regurgitation:** Though the murmur is heard at left side at tricuspid area. In cases of PAH with RVH. The murmur may be heard at apex. It increases on inspiration.

Ejection Systolic Murmurs

i. **HOCM:** An ejection systolic murmur at cardiac apex and in left 3rd and 4th space it increases by standing.

ii. In advanced cases of **AS in old people**, with the dilatation of aorta ejection systolic murmur is heard over apex though it is best heard at LPS edge (Gallavardin effect).

Significant of Systolic Murmur Over Precordium (Fig. 4.15)

Systolic murmur is produced by turbulence to blood flow in systole at cardiac valves or due to pressure difference between two sides of heart chambers (L).

In congenital defects: Like VSD, ASD.

Systolic murmur over the precordium is graded in following grades to assess the severity of lesion.

Grade I	Not heard at 1st exam, heard in quiet surrounding
Grade II	Faint murmur which is heard when stethoscope first applied to chest wall.
Grade III	Murmur easily heard. No thrill
Grade IV	Systolic murmur with thrill
Grade V	Heard with one edge of stethoscope touching chest wall
Grade VI	Loud murmur heart with stethoscope little away from chest wall and above
Grade III to VI are usually due to organic causes. The site of murmur where 1st heard sound heard tells us about origins and defect causing the murmurs.	

Aortic area: Mostly ejection systolic murmur are heard due to:
1. Valvular AS (aortic stenosis)
2. Sub-valvular stenosis (as in HOCM)
3. Aortic regurgitation severe without AS
4. Aortic valve thickening (severe atherosclerosis)
5. MR due to PMD (papillary muscle dysfunction of MV)

Pulmonary area: Systolic murmur
1. In younger 50% can be innocent up to L grade III
2. Valvular pulmonary stenosis
3. ASD (atrial septal defect)
4. Pulmonary hypertension
5. IDPA (idiopathic dilatation of pulmonary artery that is associated with click).

Systolic murmur at left 3rd and 4th space (Erb area) (Fig. 4.9)
1. Ejection murmur not common except AS, when referred from aortic area.
2. Tetralogy of Fallot
3. Small VSD/medium VSD which has PSM and in large VSD
4. Tricuspid stenosis
5. Coarctation of aorta.

Murmur at mitral area (Fig. 4.16)
1. MR (mitral regurgitation), RHD
2. Referred from aortic area in severe AS
3. MVP
4. IHD, PMD
5. Dilated ring—cardiomyopathies with dilated LV
6. Connective tissue disorders
7. SLE, rheumatoid arthritis?
8. Ankylosing spondylitis.

Section 2

Electrocardiographic Recording

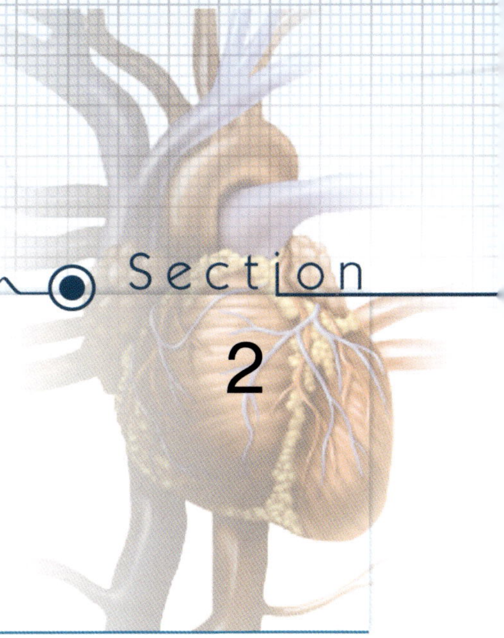

Chapter 5

ECG (Electrocardiography) of Non-IHD Cases

ECG recording during examination of heart is very common now and is almost a part of clinical examination. Most practicing doctors even at MBBS level have an ECG machine, or get it done for required cardiac cases or any patient above age of 40–50 years. So it is important to discuss ECG's role in clinical examination.

ECG Examination is Indicated in Patients of

1. **Chest pain** suspected IHD–to diagnose at earliest, angina pectoris/acute MI (myocardial infarction).
2. **Hypertension**-BP more than 139/89 mm Hg.
3. Case of **rheumatic fever** with or without valvular involvement.
4. Case of **COPD** or bronchial asthma.
5. Children with a history of **cyanosis** or with a **cardiac murmur**.
6. All established cases of **congenital heart disease**.
7. In any case of **cerebral stroke**, old or fresh.
8. History of **syncope**—to exclude AV block or CHB (complete heart block).
9. History of **acute palpitations**.
10. Any case of an **irregularly irregular pulse**.
11. History of missed beat often or as **paired VPC**.
12. History of **cardiac arrest** recovered.
13. Patient on a **pacemaker or requiring AICD implantation**.
14. **Bradycardia** or **persistent tachycardia** cases.
15. **LVF** or **CCF**.
16. Suspected **cardiac drug side effects in cases, having been** used for a long time like beta blockers or amlodipine.
17. **Before any planned surgery** above 40 years.
18. As a part of an evaluation of **medical fitness for recruitment of soldiers** in the Armed forces or **police services**.
19. Family history of **IHD** or **hypertension** or **diabetes mellitus**, or any other heart disease.
20. Medical examination before **patient's insurance** above 40 years.

ECG Recording

ECG is recording of electrical activity in cardiac muscle on contraction and relaxation. This electrical activity is converted by a powerful galvanometer in an ECG machine from electrical signals of heart to waveforms to be recorded on moving paper for review by doctors. The myocardial contraction and relaxation are also called depolarisation and repolarisation based on movement of sodium and potassium ions across each muscle cell wall (Fig. 5.1).

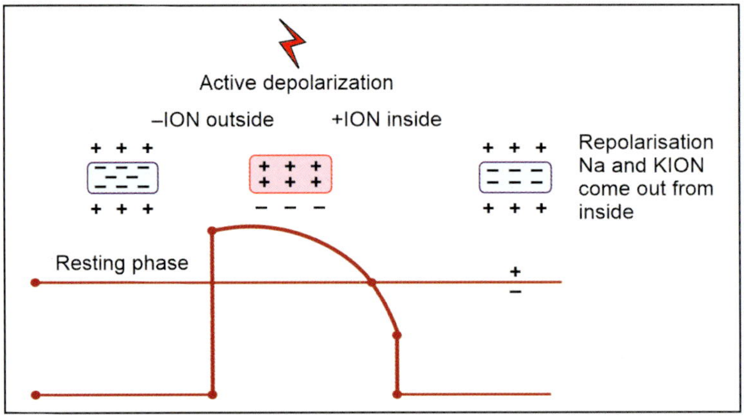

Fig. 5.1: Diagrammatic electromyogram of single myocardial cell

Ionic movements, across a single heart muscle fibre wall in depolarisation and repolarisation produce electric gradient. Total of these electric gradients is ECG signals picked up by different leads is ECG.

Electrical Activity of Heart (Fig. 5.2)

It originates in three areas of the heart:

1. Cardiac pacemaker cells at SA node, in right atrium.
2. Specialised conduction tissues—AV node–His bundle and its branches and Purkinje fibres up to ventricular muscles.
3. Heart muscle itself.

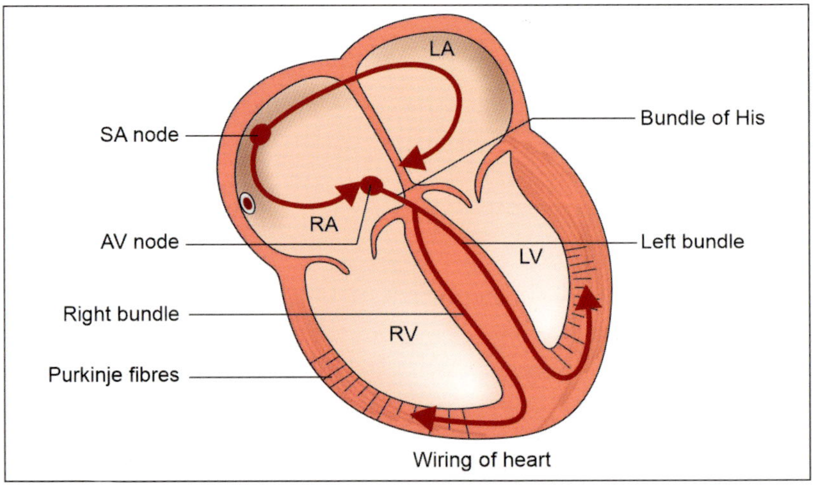

Fig. 5.2: Normal cardiac impulse passage from SA node via AV node to the ventricle (LV and RV)

Excitation or depolarisation usually begins in the SA node. It spreads as a wave through both the atria muscles. It cannot go to ventricles directly as the atria are insulated from ventricles. It comes to AV node where its speed slows down, then passes through the bundle of His and its branches (right and left) and finally into Purkinje fibres in both ventricles. Different areas of the heart are depolarised at different speeds and at different times.

Depolarisation Speed

Atrial muscle: 1 meter per second
AV node: 0.2 meter per second
His bundle and branches: 4.0 meters per second
Ventricular muscle: 0.15 meter per second.

The depolarisation wave spreads from the endocardium to the epicardium. Repolarisation wave occurs after some delay, during which time cardiac action potential comes to resting level. Then repolarisation current starts much slower from epicardium to endocardium, taking more time.

Wave Forms of ECG

P wave of ECG represents atrial depolarisation, QRS represents ventricular depolarization, ST segment represents isoelectric phase, T wave (more slower and broader than QRS) represents repolarisation.

Recording Leads

Bipolar limb leads (Fig. 5.3a and b) } in a vertical plane
Augmented unipolar limb leads (Fig. 5.4a and b) } in a vertical plane
Chest leads in a horizontal plane (Fig. 5.5a and b).

All leads both horizontal and frontal plane are diagrammatically shown in Fig. 5.6.

ECG Leads (Figs 5.3a to 5.6)

With 6 pairs of lead, 12 leads, each patient is connected to the ECG machine. They conduct the electrical charges in different parts of heart to ECG machine which as mentioned previously with the help of a powerful galvanometer converts it into different waveforms recorded on ECG paper moving at a speed of 25 mm per second.

ECG Paper Special (Fig. 5.7)

A graph paper strip available in rolled-up bundle is fitted in the ECG machine. This paper has vertical and horizontal lines 1 mm apart. Horizontal axis represents time; vertical axis represents amplitude of ECG wave. The heavy black lines are 5 mm apart in both planes. The thin lines of small square are 0.04 millisecond apart. Five small squares are 1 mm × 1 mm, and big squares are 5 mm × 5 mm apart (Fig. 5.8).

Normal ECG Record (Figs 5.8 and 5.9)

It represents different waves of different amplitude and intervals as shown in an enlarged format of an ECG. Each wave is described below. The duration of ECG waves is measured along the horizontal axis and voltage on a vertical axis. ECG is recorded at a speed of 25 mm per second. With one small square one mm represents 0.04 second or 40 milliseconds. A big square on paper 5 mm being equivalent to 0.20 or 200 milliseconds. Standardised ECG paper records the ECG of each lead for 10 seconds.

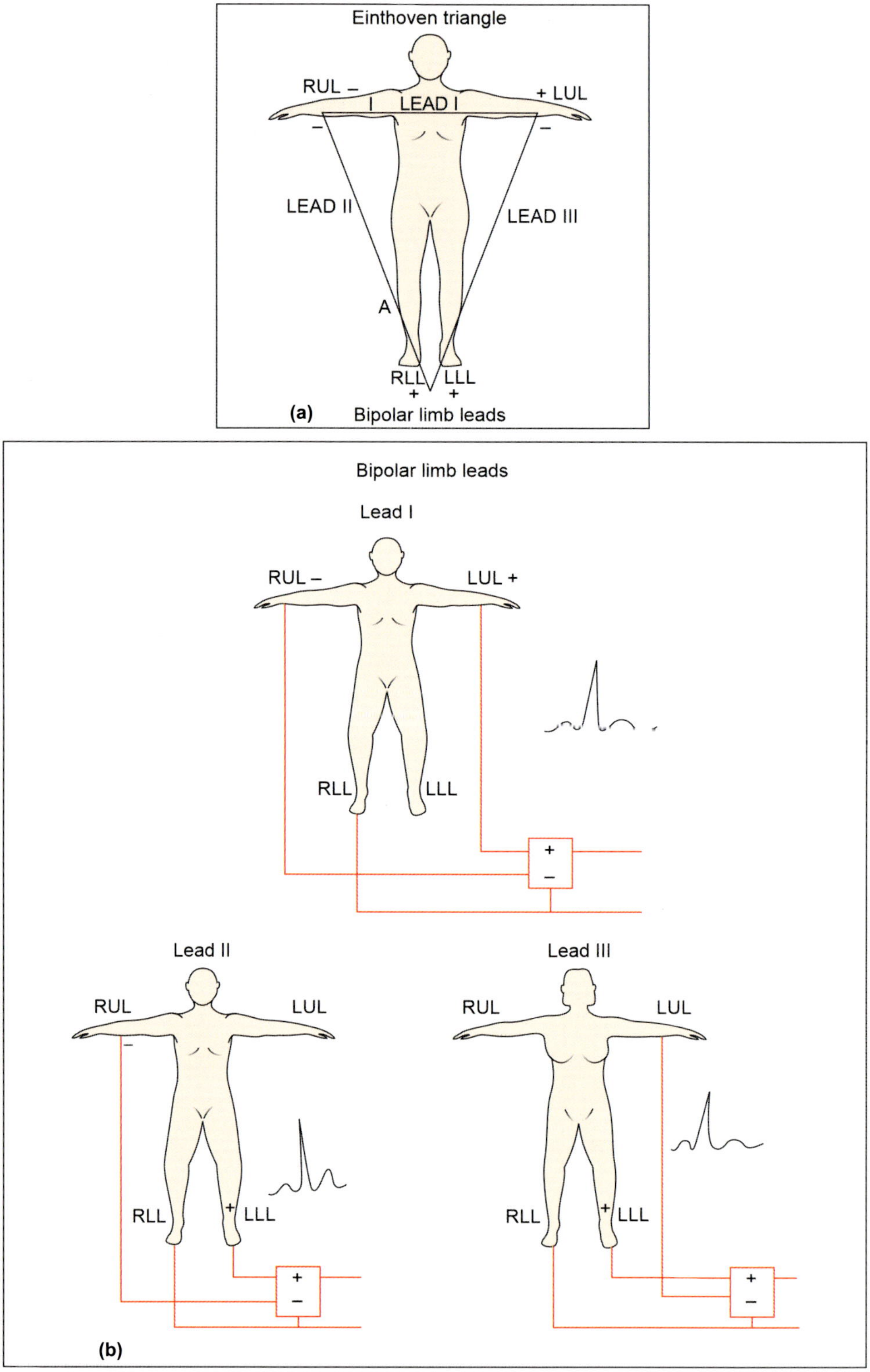

Fig. 5.3a and b: Bipolar limb leads

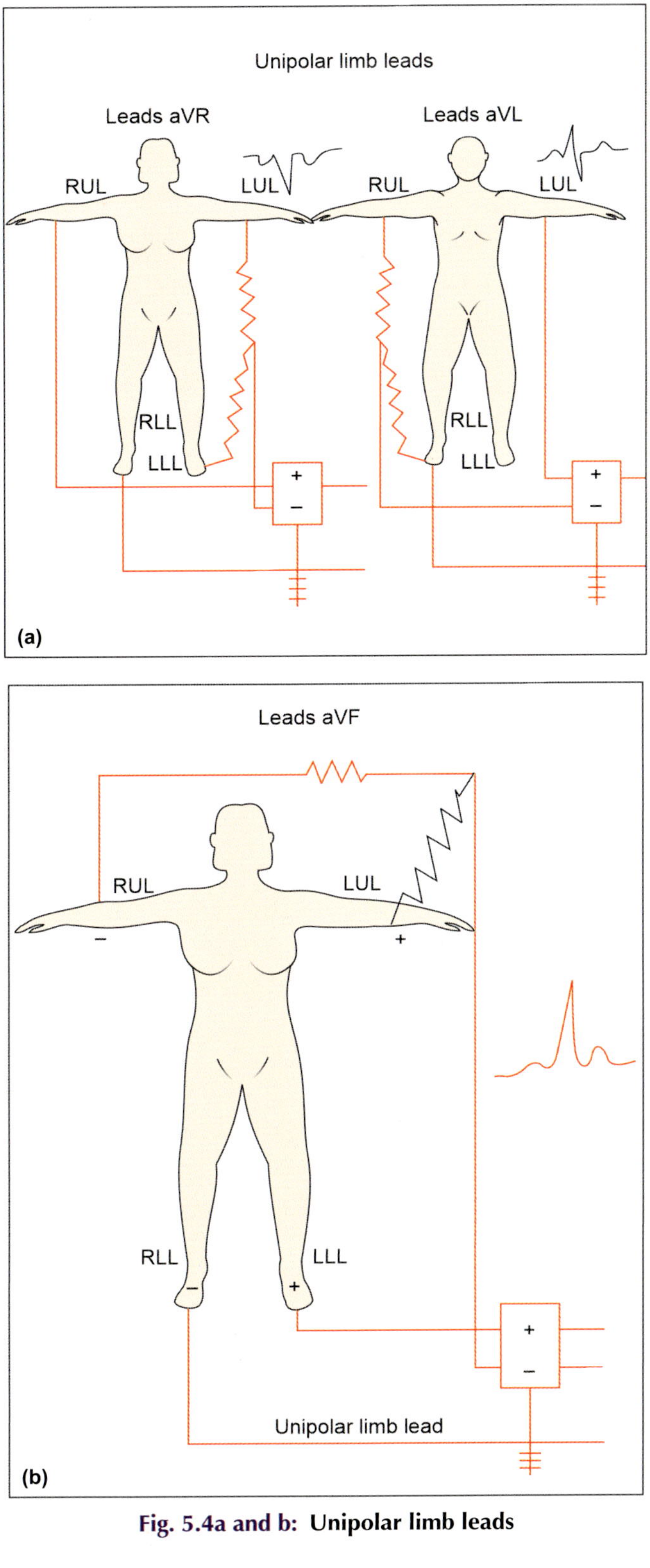

Fig. 5.4a and b: Unipolar limb leads

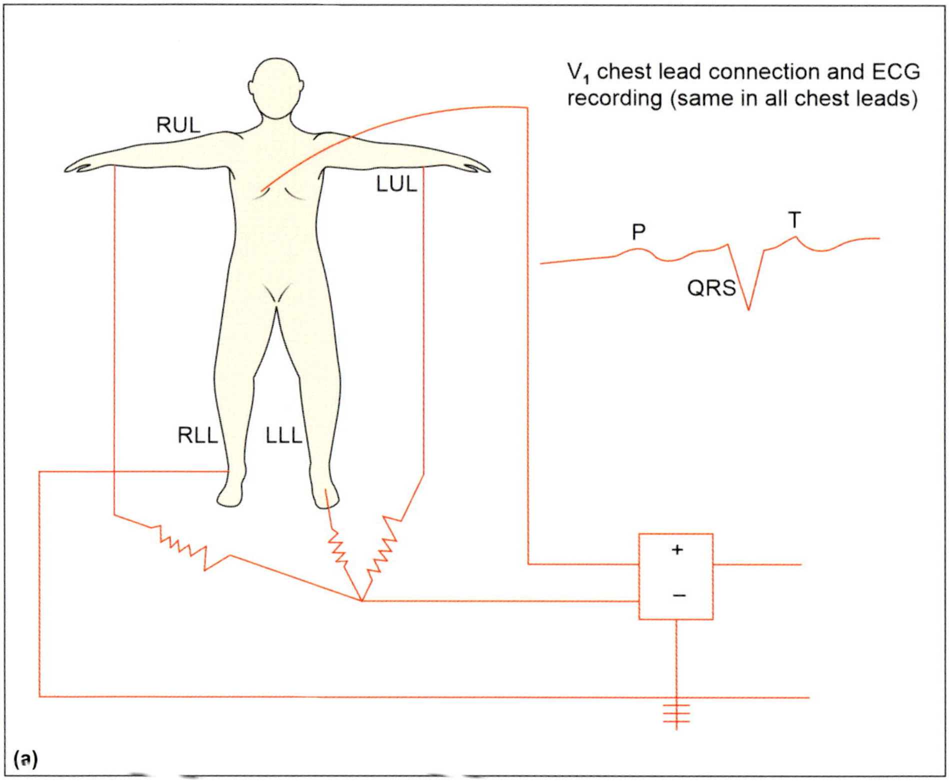

Lead	*+ve input*	*–ve input*
Bipolar limb lead		
I	LA	RA
II	LL	RA
III	LL	LA
Augmented unipolar limb leads		
aVR	RA	LA + LL
aVL	LA	RA + LL
aVF	LL	LA + RA
Precordial leads		
V_1	Right sternal margin 4th space	Wilson central terminal (LA + RA + LL)
V_2	Left sternal margin 4th space	Do
V_3	Midway between V_2 and V_4	Do
V_4	Left midclavicular line 5th IC space	Do
V_5	Left anterior axillary line in same plane as V_4	Do
V_6	Left midaxillary line in same plane as V_4	Do
LA—left arm; RA—right arm; LL—left leg		

(b)

5

Fig. 5.5a and b: (a) Basic electrogenesis of chest lead, (b) placement of six pair of leads for ECG recording

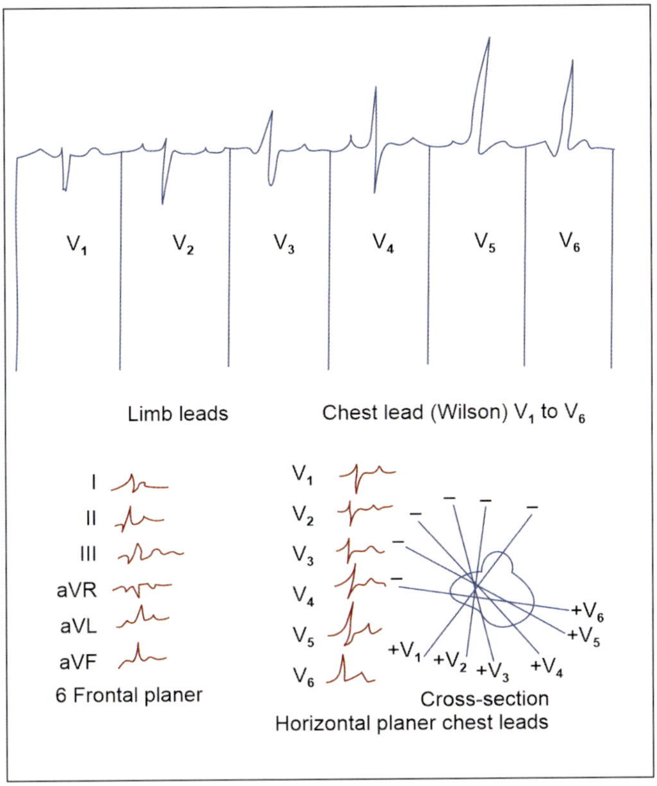

Fig. 5.6: Placement of six pair of leads for ECG recording

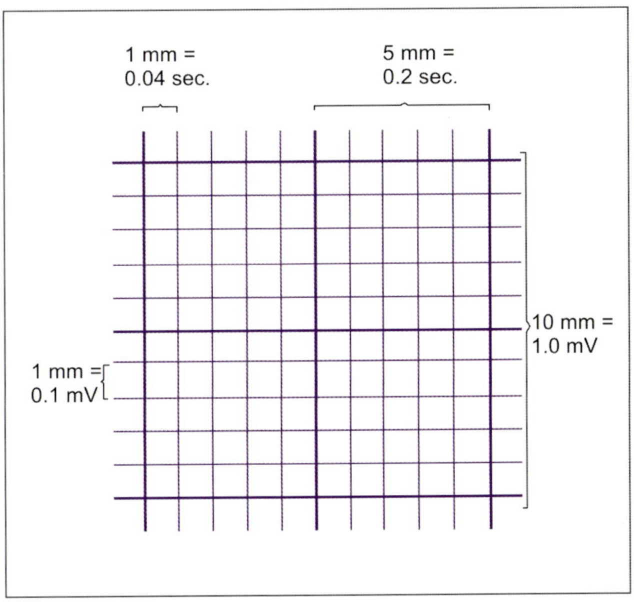

Fig. 5.7: ECG recording paper: The time interval in thin vertical grid lines are applicable for standard paper speed of 25 mm per sec for each small square in horizontal planes 0.04 sec and a big square of 5 small square is = 0.20 sec. Similarly, interval between the thin lines on the vertical axis is 0.1 mV = 1 mm and a big square of thick black line is 5 mm

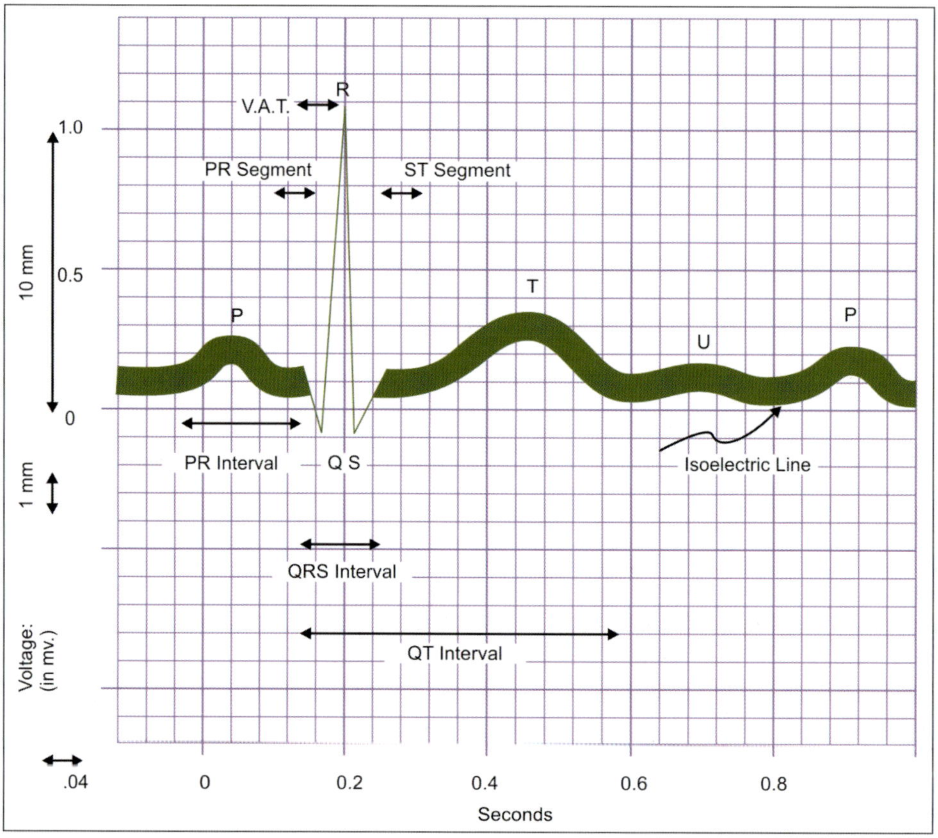

Fig. 5.8: Normal ECG calibrated intervals and segments at 100 mm per second and ECG wave format

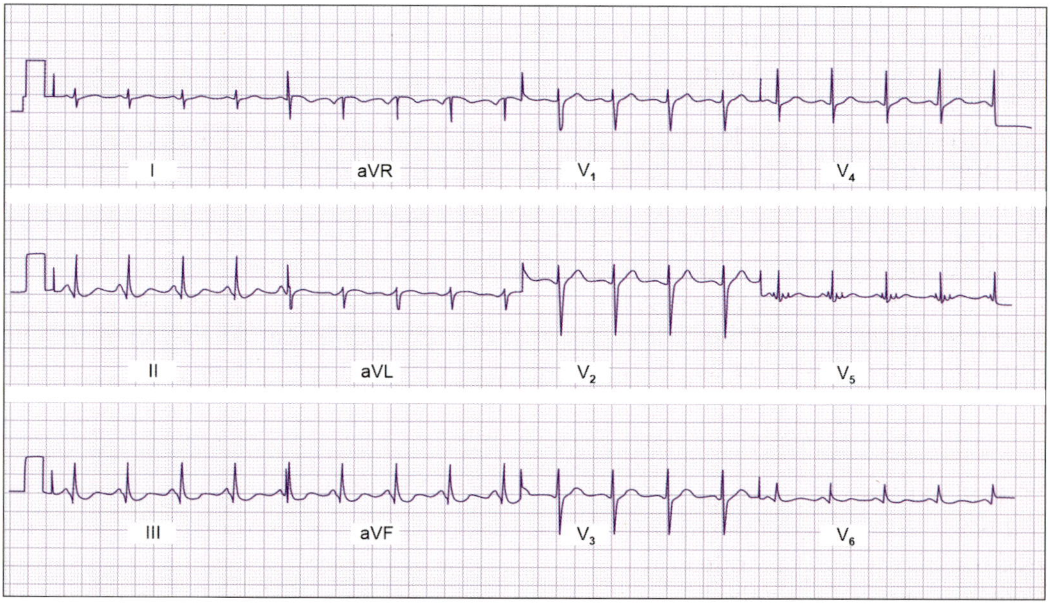

Fig. 5.9: Normal ECG leads on 3 channel monitor; Normal AQRS –30° to +110°

Technically Good ECG Recording

Good recorded ECG is exemplified by standardisation signals of 10 mm voltage on ECG paper with a properly applied pressure of stylus shown on the corner of a signal at a right angle. Overdamped stylus with more pressure will show complexes of low voltage. The light stylish records artificially high voltage waves. Each lead should have at least 3 ECG complexes.

ECG Waveforms (Figs 5.8 and 5.9)

Waves over 5 millimetre amplitude written in capital letters QRS, waves less than 5 millimetres as qrs. The leads are always labelled beginning with a P wave. P wave is produced by atrial depolarisation producing contraction of both atria. Initial negative deflection from ventricular depolarisation produces a q wave. It precedes first positive deflection of ventricular depolarisation, i.e. R wave. Q wave if less than 5 millimetres is written as q wave. If more than 5 millimetres and more than 25% of next R wave then it is pathological and usually a sign of myocardial infarction written as Q wave. R wave is the first positive deflection if more than 5 mm. If less than 5 millimetres written as r wave. It is due to ventricular depolarisation, the depolarisation current moving from endocardium to epicardium causes the deflection of wave in ECG paper as upwords. S wave is first negative deflection of ventricular depolarisation following R wave. If S wave less than 5 mm, it is written as s wave.

T wave: Deflection is produced by ventricular repolarisation when the current moves from the epicardium to the endocardium in the heart.

U wave: It is an upwards deflection seen sometimes in few ECG leads following T waves but before the next P wave. It is not seen in all the leads and also in all the patients. Mostly seen in V_1, V_2 and V_3. U wave is a sign of hypokalaemia.

Normal Segment in ECG

PR segment begins from the P wave to the beginning of QRS complex. It measures AV conduction time including conduction delay at AV node 0.07 second and passage of impulse through a bundle of His and its branches to the onset of ventricular depolarisation. Normal PR segment measures 0.12–0.20 seconds, mostly is isoelectric and best measured in lead II and lead VI. Normally athletes can have PR intervals up to 0.22 milliseconds.

ST segment begins from end of QRS at J point to the beginning of T wave. It is isoelectric but normally may be elevated with concavity upwards by 2 mm or depressed by 0.5 mm in lead V_1, V_2, or V_3 especially in women up to the age of 40 years. This change is seen in all the ECGs of the patient taken at any time, unlike the ST elevation seen in acute MI. The elevation or depression is measured in relation to TP segment from the end of T wave to the beginning of P wave.

ECG Intervals

RR interval indicates a distance between successive R-wave, measured from the peak of R wave to the peak of the next R wave. Distance varies with heart rate and it can be used for measuring heart rate. If we divide 300 by a number of big squares between two R waves, for example, 5 the heart rate is 60 per minute. If we divide 1500 by a number of small squares, for example, 25, between the two R waves, the heart rate is also 60.

Cardiac Axis

The cardiac axis is the mean direction of the vectors of all electrical forces at a particular place in the vertical plane (Fig. 5.10). Its measurements are of considerable value in fine-tuning the diagnosis of myocardial diseases by ECG. It is measured by three practical methods at bedside.

Methods of Measurement of Cardiac Axis

1. Quadrant method of using lead I and lead aVF.

Predominant positive QRS in Lead I and predominant negative in Lead aVF means left cardiac axis, i.e. beyond –30° (left axis deviation). Positive QRS in Lead I and lead aVF means **normal** axis –30° to +110°. Negative lead I and positive lead aVF mean right axis (+110 to +150) right axis indeterminate axis between is beyond +150° to upper right quadrant (Fig. 5.11).

2. Axis determination by a perpendicular method

Please look at the lead in which QRS is biphasic. Axis in lead which is perpendicular to this lead, e.g. biphasic in Lead II then axis is 60 degrees. This means QRS axis is perpendicular to lead with equiphasic or small QRS complex. For example, if the QRS is equiphasic in lead II, the QRS axis must be perpendicular to the axis of lead II (Table 5.1 and Fig. 5.12).

Table 5.1: Axis determination by the perpendicular method

Leads with biphasic QRS	*QRS axis in frontal plane*
I (0°)	+90° or –90°
II (+60°)	–30° or +150°
III (+120°)	+30° or –150°
aVR (–150°)	+120° or –60°
aVL (–30°)	+60° or –120°
aVF (+90°)	0° or +180°

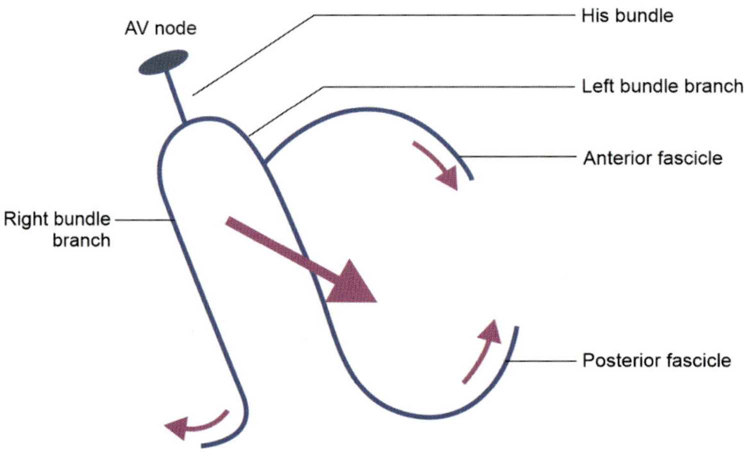

5

Fig. 5.10: Normal vector direction: Mean frontal QRS axis normal –30° to +110°. This is the mean direction of LV depolarising vector in 6 leads (I to AVF) that lie in the frontal plane of the heart at the right angle of lead in which Q ↔ RS deflection is least pronounced

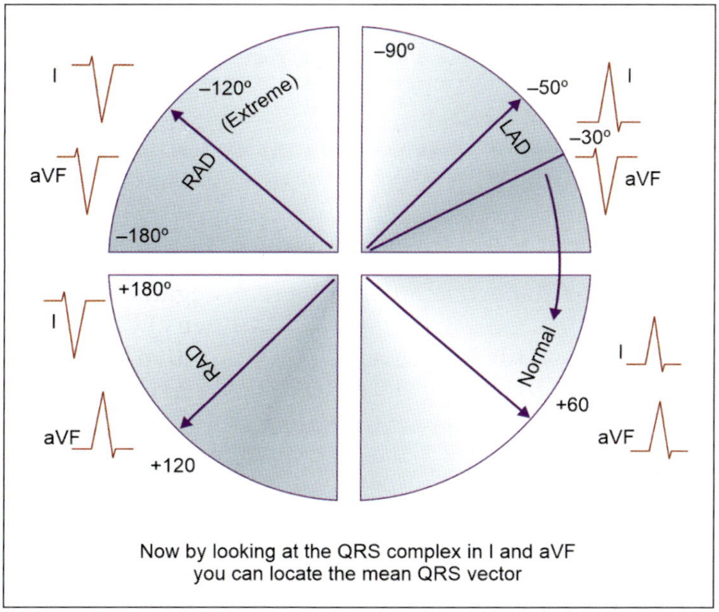

Now by looking at the QRS complex in I and aVF, you can locate the mean QRS vector.

Fig. 5.11: Quadrant method of axis determination in frontal plane

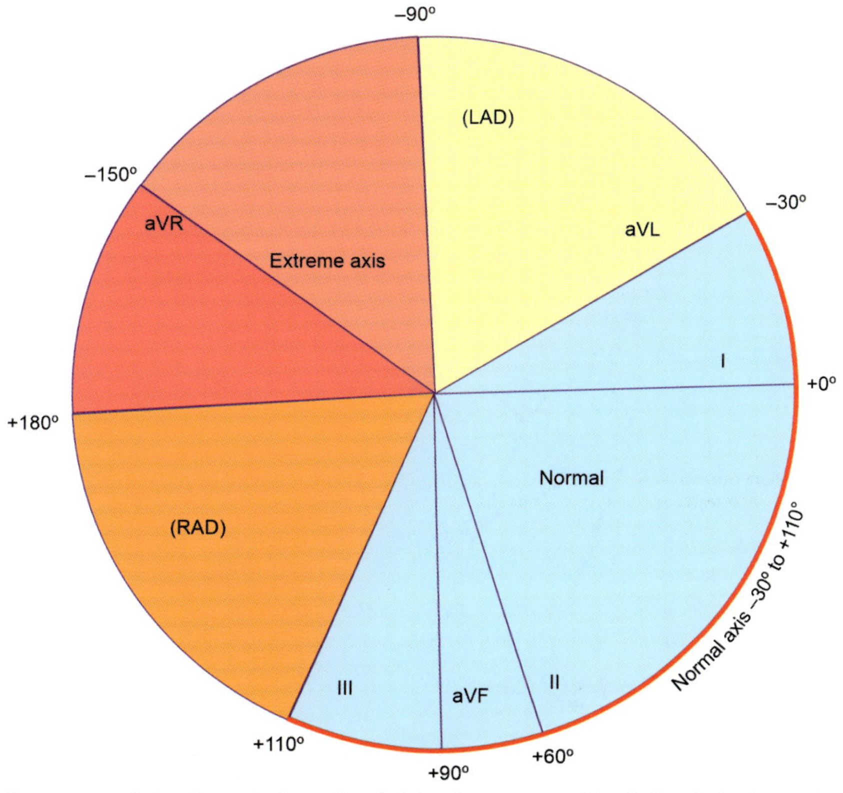

Fig. 5.12: Axis in (frontal plane) its division in areas used in daily clinical practice

5

3. **Objective calculation of axis by simple method** (Fig. 5.13)

- Generally the axis of leads I and aVF is used to calculate the axis of the QRS complex. For this net deflection of QRS in each lead is calculated by subtracting deflection of Q wave from deflection of R wave (e.g. if in lead I, Q wave measures three small squares and R–wave height is six small squares, the net deflection is +3).
- Net positive deflection in lead I is plotted on the left side and net positive in lead aVF is plotted upward. Perpendiculars from these points are drawn and then a line is drawn from centre to the intersection of perpendiculars. This represents the axis of QRS complex.
- The normal QRS axis is –30° to +110°.

Table 5.2: Common causes of axis deviation

Left axis deviation (LAD)	*Right axis deviation (RAD)*
• Left bundle branch block	• Right ventricular hypertrophy
• Inferior wall myocardial infarction	• Chronic obstructive airway disease
• Hypertrophic cardiomyopathy	• Atrial septal defect (ostium secundum types)
• Left ventricular hypertrophy	
• Atrial septal defect (ostium primum type)	

Electrocardiograph Report (Fig. 5.9)

In the previous paragraph different waveforms segments and intervals of normal ECG, their electrogenesis and variations have been described separately. When we concentrate on an ECG one should use the following protocol to give its report so that no event is missed in its interpretation. **Name of patient, age, sex, date, time, serial number of ECG, hospital/clinic OPD/IPD registration number of patients and give details of all the important positive and negative waves besides intervals, axis, rate,**

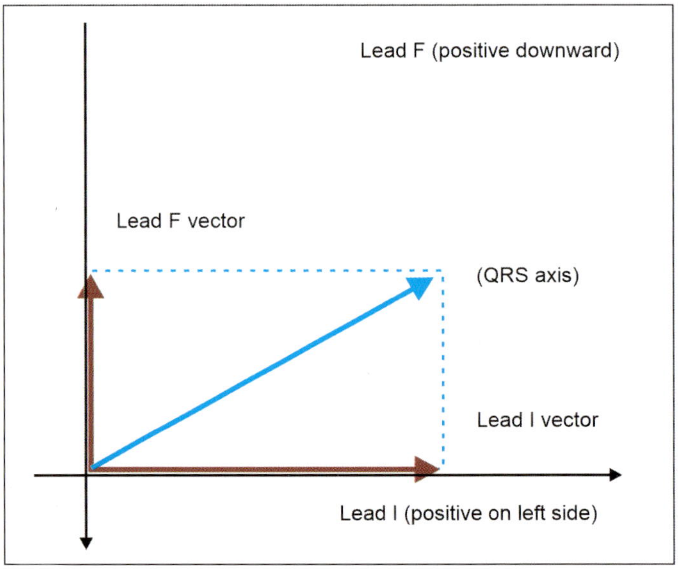

Fig. 5.13: Calculation of QRS axis

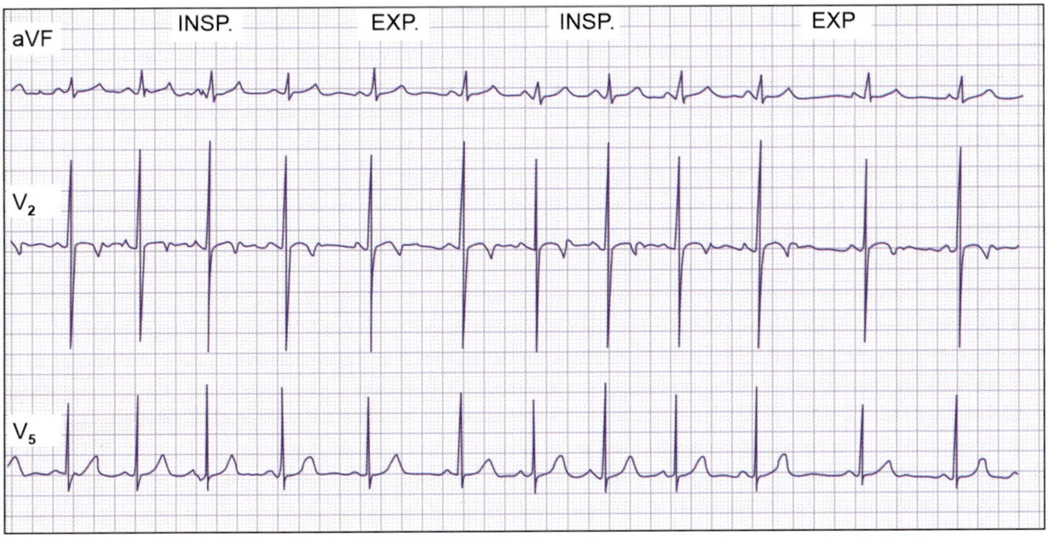

Fig. 5.13: Sinus arrhythmia: It is a normal variation of heart rate. In inspiration, heart rate increases due to a decrease in the vagal inhibitory effect on the SA node, thereby increase in the heart rate. The reverse happens during expiration so the heart rate decreases in expiration. This vagal effect on the SA node disappears in old age and in autonomic neuropathy. No change in the shape of P-wave and the P-R interval remains constant.

rhythm, ST segment changes, QRS and T waves changes in the reported ECG and finally the ECG diagnosis.

1. **Rate:** Normal rate is 60–100 per minute except in professional athletes it can be 45 to 50 per minute due to high vagal tone. RR interval method as described earlier is used to measure heart rate. Sympathetic stimulation increases heart rate while parasympathetic stimulation decreases heart rate, i.e. vagal effect.
2. **Rhythm:** It can be **sinus rhythm**. Each P wave is followed by QRS and T wave. But sometimes PR interval is not constant. In such cases, we count RR interval in 6 seconds of ECG recorded on a long rhythm strip of lead II or V_1 and multiply it by 10 to get heart rate per minute. In normal sinus rhythm P wave is positive in lead I, II, aVF, aVL, V_2–V_6 and biphasic in V_1, III, negative aVR. **Best leads to study P wave are lead II or V_1.**

ECG Abnormalities in Rate and Rhythm

Sinus arrhythmia: In a normal person heart rate increases in inspiration and decreases in expiration, a difference of 10% in RR interval. In one-third of young people it is present, it is called respiratory sinus arrhythmia. It is a normal variation (Fig. 5.13a).

Sinus tachycardia (Fig. 5.14): It is when the heart rate is more than 100 per minute. Normally with sympathetic stimulation, it can go up to 180 to 200 per minute in healthy young adults during maximum exercise. It has p wave followed by QRS wave. Above 70 years it can go maximum up to 140–150 per minute. P wave may merge with the preceding T wave. Common causes are **anxiety, physical exertion, pain, sympathomimetic drugs like dopamine, epinephrine, cocaine derived drugs and anticholinergic drugs like atropine. Also, heart rate is increased in fever, septic shock,**

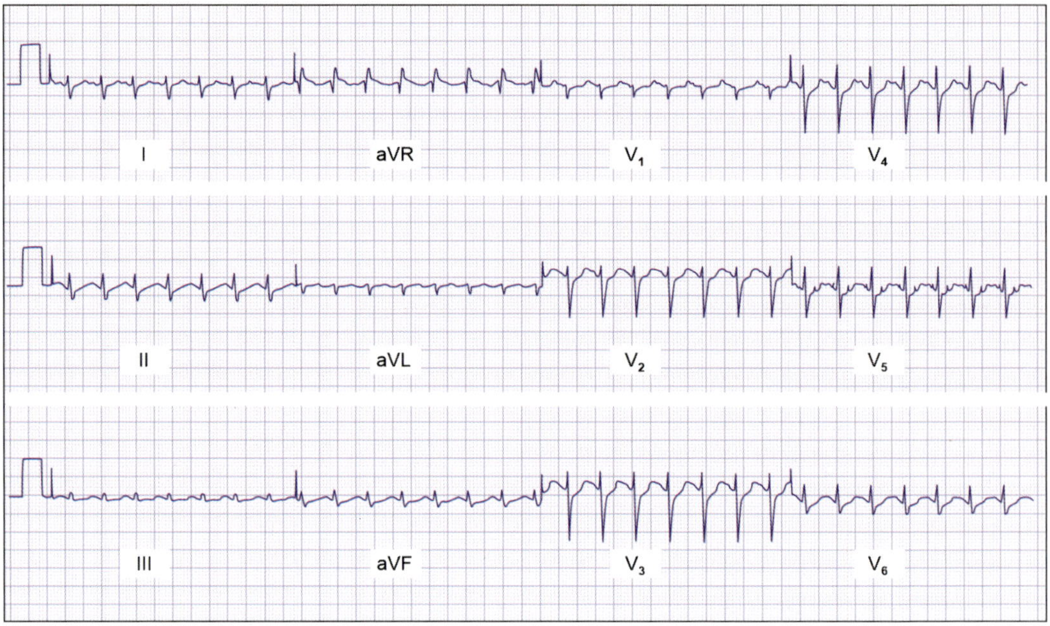

Fig. 5.14: Sinus tachycardia: In sinus tachycardia sometimes rapid upsloping ST segment ↓ seen in normal person heart rate 180 per minute

LVF, CCF, hyperthyroidism, ACS (acute coronary syndrome). Alcohol intoxication, excess smoking (more than 10 cigarettes per day), too much coffee or tea (more than 6 cups per day) also cause sinus tachycardia.

Sinus bradycardia (Fig. 5.15): It is when the heart rate is less than 60 per minute. In ECG P wave followed by QRS is seen in those with high vagal tone, like in athletes. It can go down to 50 per minute. Common causes are normal in athletes while sleeping, **digoxin** and drugs increasing vagal tone, drugs decreasing sympathetic tone like beta-blockers, calcium channel blockers, diltiazem and verapamil, hypothyroidism, hyperkalaemia (serum potassium more than 6 mEq per litre), increased ICP (Intracranial pressure) (Fig. 5.16), SSS (sick sinus syndrome), in elderly especially, tight neck tie, which causes pressure on carotid sinus in the neck.

Sinus Node Related Arrhythmias

Ischaemia or age-related degenerative changes in the sinus node fails to initiate cardiac impulse, so no atrial contraction and no P wave or QRS seen in ECG for one or two consecutive heartbeats, we call it **sinus pause. It can be of two types:**

a. **Sinus block** occurs when entire PQRS is absent, but PP interval during sinus block is multiple of normal PP interval—SA block (Fig. 5.17).
b. **Sinus arrest** (Fig. 5.18a and b) occurs when sinus activity is lost for more than 3 seconds. PP interval during sinus arrest is not multiple of normal PP interval. In sinus arrest, patient can feel dizzy or may lose consciousness for a short-time till normal cardiac activity starts. For sinus arrest we may require immediately TPM (temporary pacemaker) followed by bipolar PPM (permanent pacemaker), an atrial pacing lead and other ventricular pacing lead. Post-PPM ECG shows pacing spikes (Fig. 5.19).

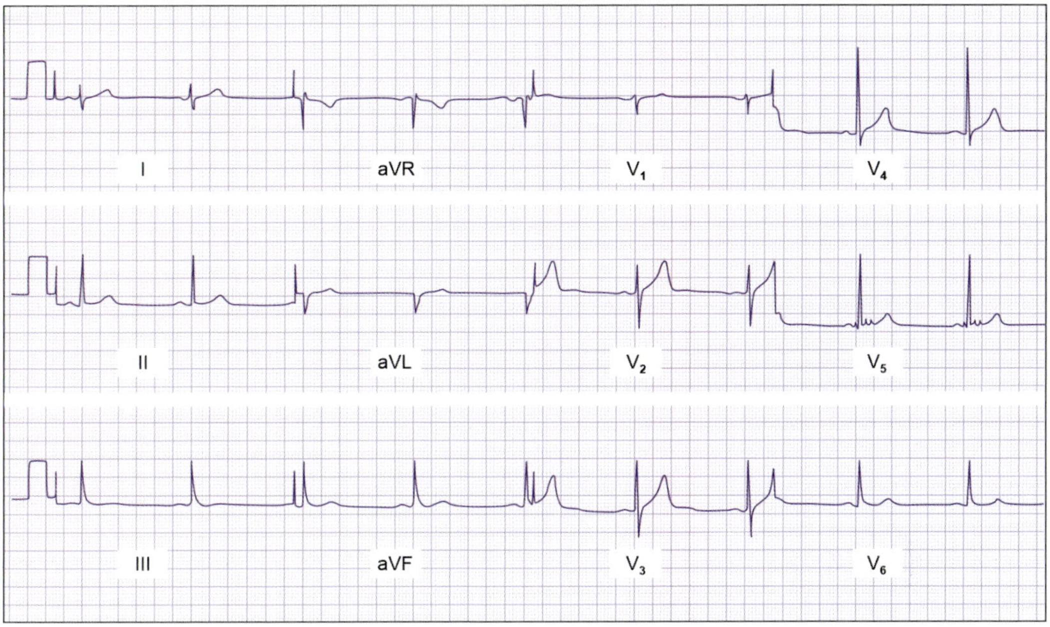

Fig. 5.15: Sinus bradycardia: Heart rate 50 per minute, all complexes are normal

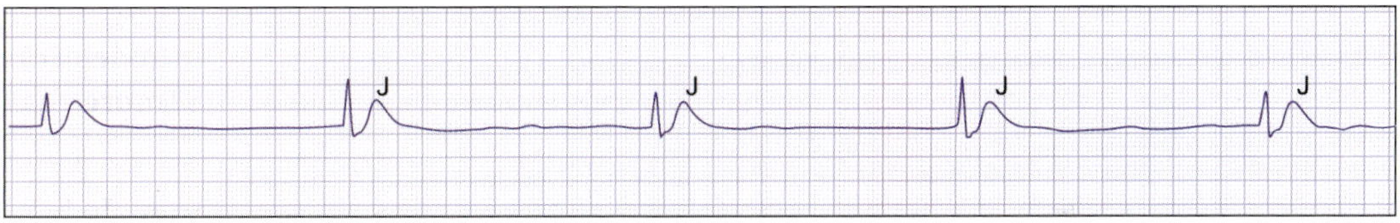

Fig. 5.16: Heart rate 15 per minute prominent J wave of Osborn raised intracranial tension

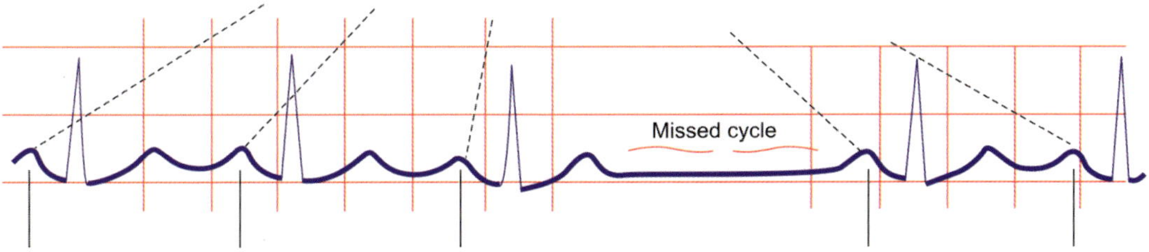

Fig. 5.17: SA (Node) block causes the pacemaker to temporarily stop for at least one cycle, but then the pacemaker resumes the pacing activity. **Diagrammatic for teaching**

Atrial Premature Beat or Complex (APC)

Definition: APC results from premature ectopic supraventricular impulse arising somewhere outside SA node. Also called premature atrial complex (PAC).

1. ECG shows irregular RR intervals, PAC disturbs the regularity of underlying rhythm.
2. Shape of ectopic premature P wave is different from the sinus P wave. It could be deformed, inverted, or may be attached to the preceding T wave or buried in QRS complex.

5

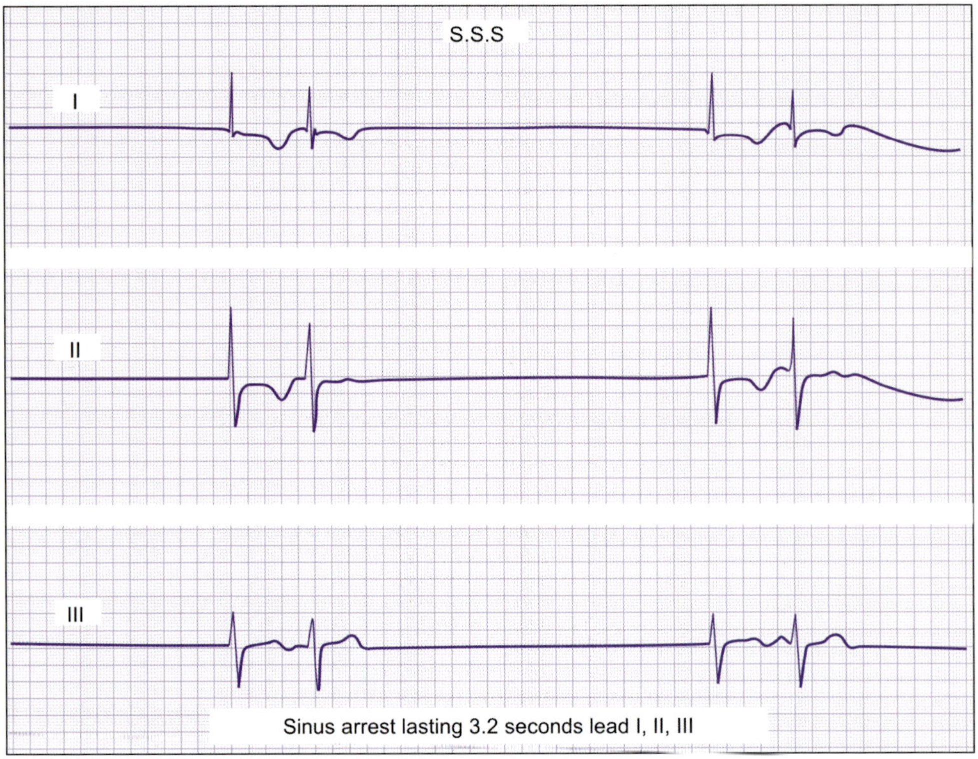

Fig. 5.18a: Sinus arrest lasting 3.2 seconds lead I, II, III

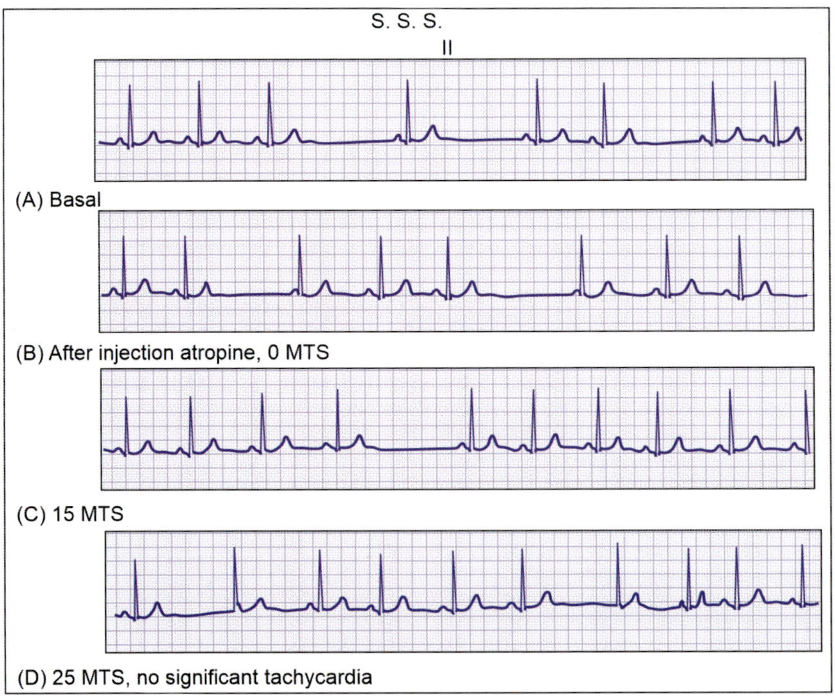

Fig. 5.18b: SSS

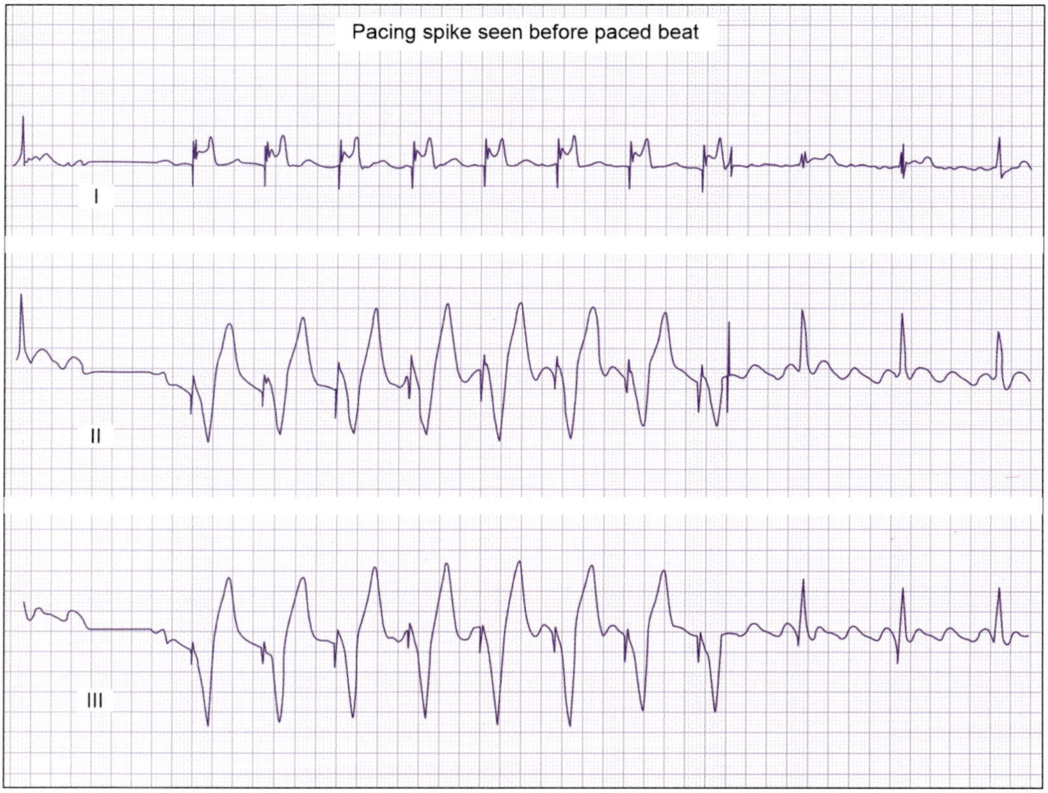

Fig. 5.19: Intermittent RV pacing L. I, II, III (pacemaker implanted)
Pacing spike clearly seen

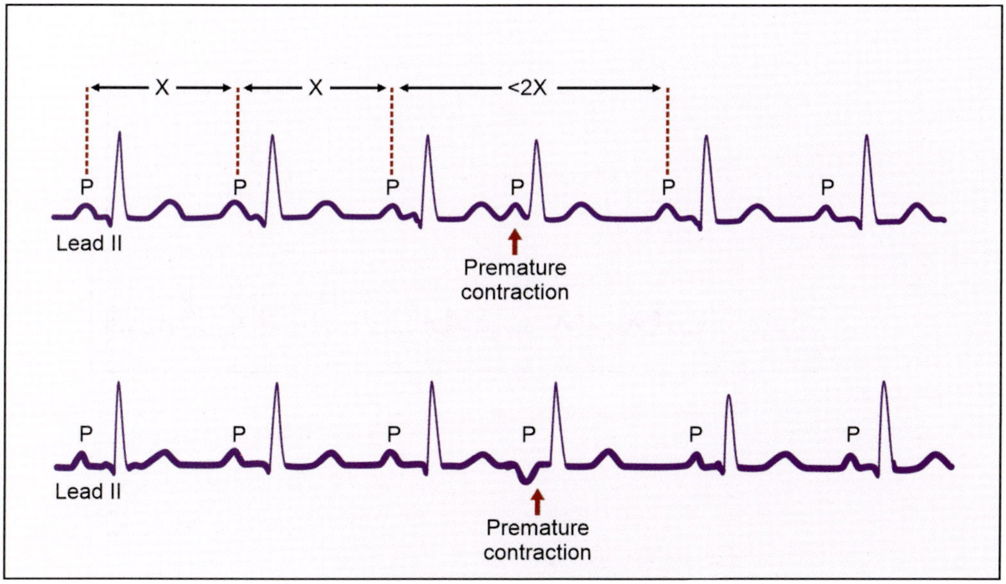

Fig. 5.19a: Premature contraction

3. PAC is invariably followed by normal QRS complex, if conducted through AV node.
4. If AV node is refractory then PAC will not be followed by QRS complex, called blocked PAC.
5. QRS complex is narrow if conduction to ventricle is undisturbed.
6. APC may be conducted with aberration if QRS is a bit wide where ventricle is yet fully repolarised from the preceding impulse.
7. Best seen in II, III, aVF, V_1.
8. When P wave is inverted in lead II, III and aVF with normal QRS its focus is in AV node close to the sinus at the root of the aorta, it is called coronary sinus rhythm, it is benign rhythm.

Causes of APC: Normal in anxiety, mental stress, excess coffee or alcohol, any heart disease like CCF, acute MI, congenital heart disease (operated), COPD, pericarditis, electrolyte disturbance like hyperkalaemia, digoxin toxicity, and hypertension.

Treatment: Find the cause. If symptomatic requires verapamil, diltiazem, excess anxiety needs beta-blocker. If sinus tachycardia persists after drug treatment, EPS (electrophysiological studies) done and irritable focus identified, then ablation of irritable focus can be done.

Paroxysmal Atrial Tachycardia (PAT)

Supraventricular rhythm originating in atria outside SA node at rate 120–250 per minute (Figs 5.20 and 5.21).

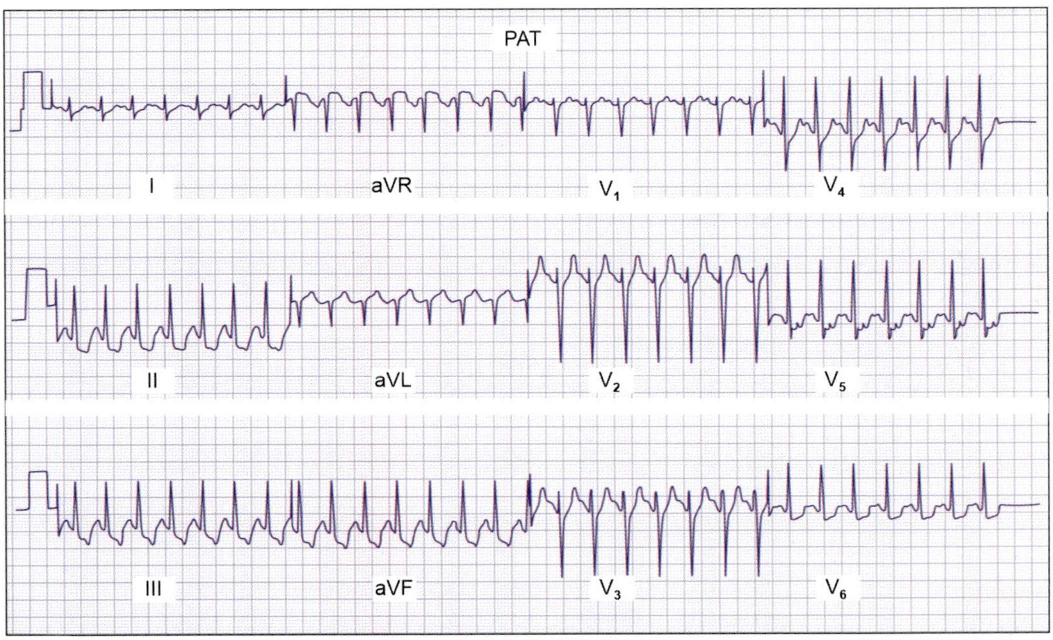

Fig. 5.20: H/R 188 per min slow upsloping ST ↓ in II, AVL, V3, V4, V6 down sloping ST in ↓ III, aVF

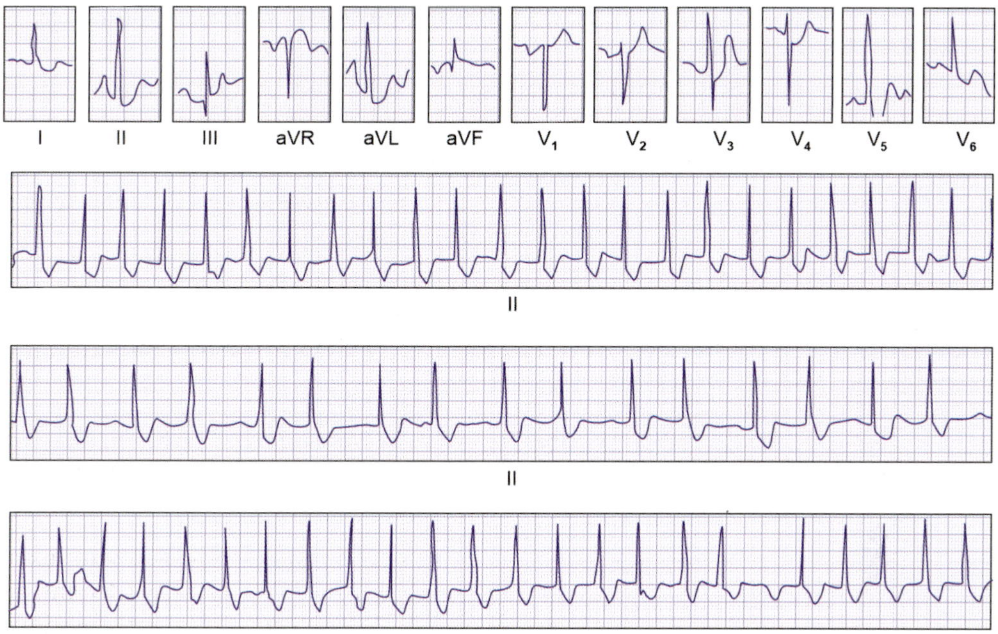

Fig. 5.21: SVT (supraventricular tachycardia) HR >160 per min constant R-R interval

Common Causes

1. RHD
2. Digitalis toxicity
3. Idiopathic
4. Hyperthyroidism
5. Post-surgery of congenital heart disease
6. Hypokalaemia
7. Hypertension
8. CCF.

ECG: Regular rhythm, PP and RR interval equal. Rate 120–250 per min. Conduction 1:1.

Rarely in digitalis toxicity, it could be 2:1 or 3:1, when called atrial tachycardia with AV block.

1. PR interval short when conduction through AV node.
2. P wave seen but has different morphological shapes.
3. Maybe on T wave, just short of T wave of preceding beat. P wave is best seen in Lead II, III, aVF, V1.
4. QRS narrow mostly.
5. PAT maybe paroxysmal 3–4 bursts lasting 30 seconds or may sustain up to 3 minutes or more.

Treatment

- No digoxin. Correct electrolyte disturbance
- Injection adenosine or diltiazem

5

- Dose: Injection **adenosine** 3 mg IV bolus through central venous line or 6 mg IV through peripheral vein bolus followed by 30 ml flush repeat 12 mg after 2 min interval.

Injection **diltiazem**-bolus 0.2 mg per kg in 2 min followed by 10 mg bolus after every 15–30 min.

Rarely DC (Direct Current) shock may be required, if patient is haemodynamically unstable.

Rarely injection **metoprolol** is required, 5 mg IV in 2 min, repeat 10 mg after 10 min, if DC shock facilities are not available as in peripheral Hospitals.

Paroxysmal Supraventricular Tachycardia (PSVT)

It comprises PAT, AVRT (atrioventricular reentrant tachycardia), AVNRT (AV nodal reentrant tachycardia).

ECG: APC initially a PSVT, AV conduction, P-QRS at the start but subsequently some beats show a QRS followed by P wave or QRS complex with imbibed P wave (invisible P wave). QRS complex can be aberrant (Fig. 5.22).

Treatment

Drugs

1. Adenosine
2. Diltiazem
3. Metoprolol
4. DC shock if BP decreases acutely give 30 joules, DC shock to be repeated at 60 joules, rarely up to 120 joules may be required, particularly in tall, hefty, broad-chested alcoholic individuals. R wave synchronized cardioversion done.
5. Electrophysiological studies for pathway elucidation may be required. If recurrent episodes of PSVT occur.

Atrial Flutter

Clinically patient has organic heart diseases like VSD, TVD (triple vessel disease) IHD, MVD (multivalvular disease), COPD, or after cardiac surgery, cardiomyopathy.

Patient feels palpitation, syncope, angina, with fast heart rate, and in CCF. Hypotension or syncope, the chances of thrombosis formation more in multivalvular diseases leading to systemic embolisation. Atria are enlarged and dilated.

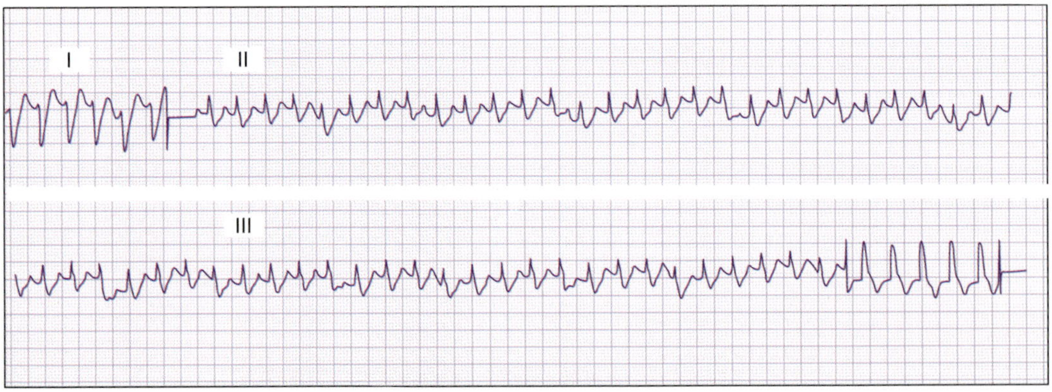

Fig. 5.22: Broad QRS tachycardia—SVT abberation

ECG: No P wave seen but sawtoothed flutter waves running irregularly along with varying RR intervals. Rarely flutter and fibrillation waves (tremor type) in some patients seen in leads II, III, aVF and V_1 (Fig. 5.23a and b).

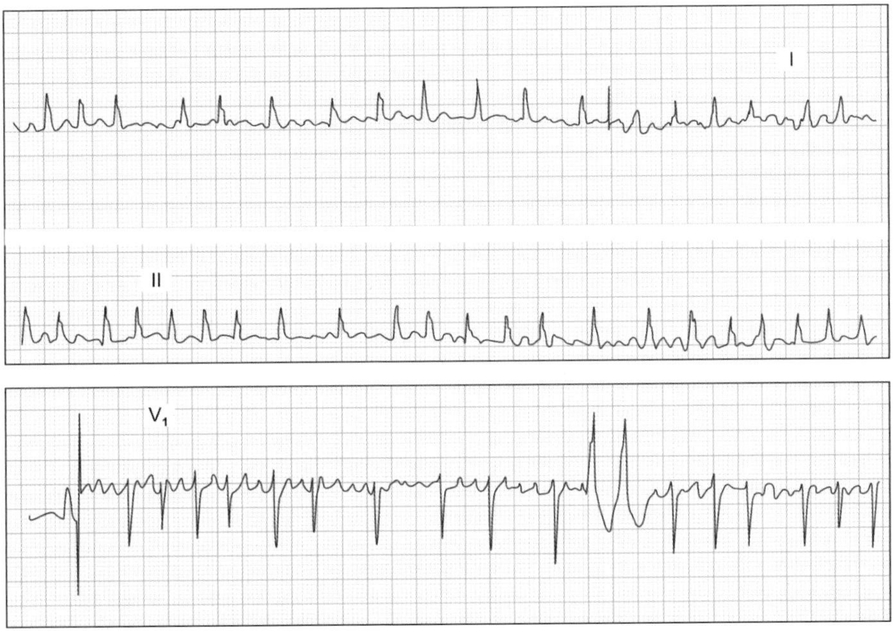

Fig. 5.23a: Atrial flutter (P wave sawtooth like) and atrial fibrillation. LII and V1

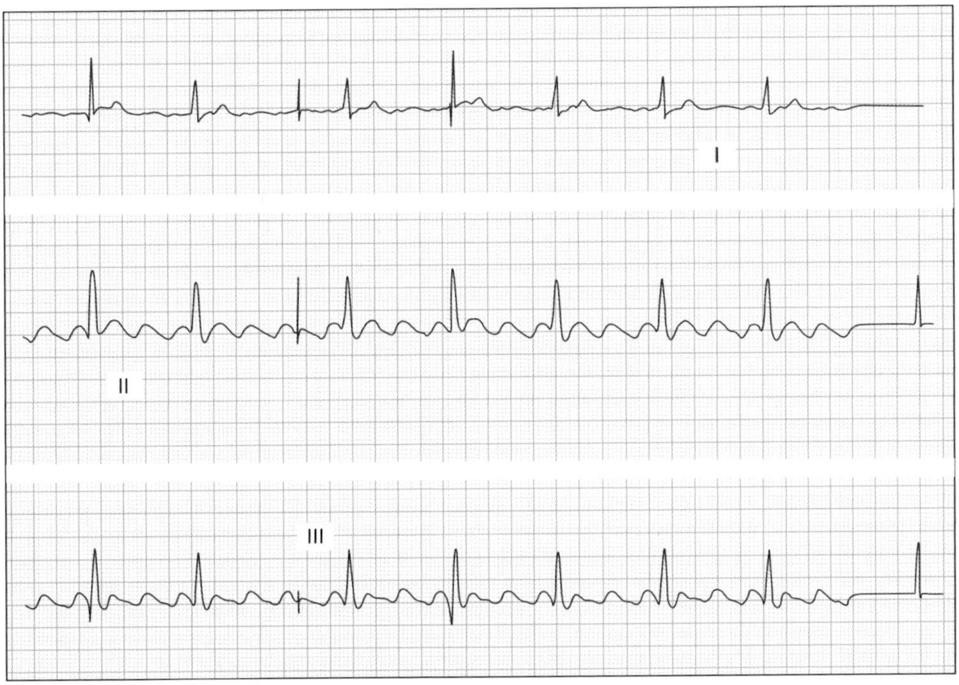

Fig. 5.23b: Atrial flutter with R-R interval not constant

Treatment

Atrial flutter rarely converts to normal on its own and even persists after drugs.

Drug Treatment

1. **Ibutulide** 0.01 mg per kg IV bolus in 10 min can be repeated after 10 min.
2. **Dofetilide** is used orally after QTC assessment and creatinine clearance estimation.
3. **Amiodarone** IV bolus and then maintenance doses (dosage to be discussed in subsequent paras) under atrial fibrillation.
4. **Anticoagulants** IV heparin in acute stage followed by clopidogrel. Keep INR 2.1–3.1. Preferably used for 24 hours before DC cardioversion is given. If previously on digoxin withhold for 24 hours. Temporary pacing done in right atrium at over 250 beats per min especially in immediate postcardiac surgery as pacing lead is already there. Now after identification of tract in right atrium by EPS (electrophysiological studies), RFA (radiofrequency ablation) is the treatment of choice for permanent cure.

Atrial Fibrillation (Fig. 5.24)

Atrial fibrillation (AF) **is one of the commonest cardiac arrhythmias**, especially in people above 50 years in India. In the Indian Heart Rhythm Society AF registry average age of AF cases in India is 54 years. It is 10 years younger than the western counterparts. RHD is seen in 47% of Indian cases. Annual mortality rate is 8% and incidence of strokes is 1%. It is commonest supraventricular tachycardia. Hypertension is commonest cause.

Mechanism

Multiple simultaneously working re-entry circuits and rotary waves in both atria are responsible for initiating and maintaining the AF.

Causes

1. RHD with MS and multivalvular disease
2. Cor pulmonale post-chronic bronchitis
3. Hypertension
4. IHD
5. ASD
6. Diabetes mellitus is a common comorbidity
7. Hyperthyroidism
8. Idiopathic also called lone AFib (atrial fibrillation)

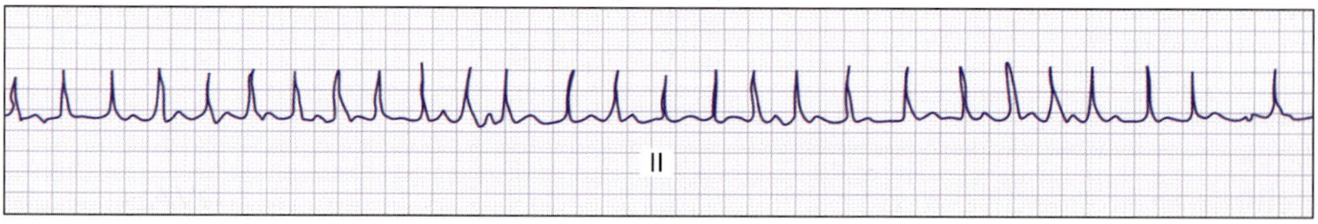

No P waves varying R R intervals rate 300 per min

Fig. 5.24: Atrial fibrillation

9. **Acute alcoholic bout: Holiday heart syndrome** especially in newly married couples when on honeymoon they compete in taking beer bottles one after the other. If not treated properly immediately by DC shock, end may be fatal. All doctors and physicians, in holiday resorts, should be aware of this medical emergency and should have DC conversion facilities available in their clinics.
10. After cardiac surgery.

Clinically-history of any coexisting morbidities as mentioned above, palpitations, effort intolerance, angina, TIA, established stroke, or CVA. Palpitations may last for minutes, hours, or days. It is classified as:

i. Paroxysmal: **AF** stops spontaneously usually within 48 hours.
ii. Persistent: If it persists for more than 7 days to months, and it fails to be terminated by drugs.

ECG rate between 90–150, irregularly irregular, BP maybe increased or decreased classical f wave in place of P wave is seen rarely. **Varying RR interval in long leads**.

Echocardiography, LV or LA dilated, or LV clot/LA clot. Cause of the heart disease identified.

Electrophysiological studies are now done at most of level III hospitals or cardiac centres to find out tract or ectopic foci near pulmonary veins entry point in LA, from where the atrial fibrillation starts.

T_3, T_4, TSH, to be exclude **thyrotoxicosis**.

Tachycardia-induced cardiomyopathy occurs in those with persistent tachycardia, at the end stage of disease.

Treatment of AF

Medical Management

i. To rate control initially—injection **ibutilide IV** 1 mg slowly over 10 min is given, it may be repeated once again to terminate AF but watch for the recurrence.
ii. Injection **diltiazem** 0.25–0.5 mg per kg over 2–5 min, repeat after 5 min and continue injection diltiazem at the rate of 0.35 mg per minute as infusion.
iii. Injection **metoprolol** 5 mg IV bolus in 5 min, repeat every 10 min up to 3 times, i.e. 15 mg and see AF is terminated or not.
iv. Injection **amiodarone** 150 mg over 10 min followed by 1 mg per min for 6 hours and continued as 0.5 mg per min infusion followed by maintenance oral dose 10 mg BD.
v. Anticoagulant for prevention of stroke, **injection heparin infusion** is best to prevent thrombosis and thromboembolic complications in RHD followed by **clopidogrel or warfarin orally**. Keep INR at 2.5 by repeated prothrombin time estimation.
vi. Patient to be kept in ICCU where ECG, BP and oximetry are continually monitored by well-trained nursing staff, medicine residents. Physician/cardiologists should visit the patient at least 4 times a day and as and when required.

Novel oral anticoagulants: Useful in cases of non-valvular, AFib in IHD, diabetes mellitus and hypertension cases. The drugs are prescribed using CHADVASC score calculated on the basis of the following risk factors: (i) age more than 65, (ii) or more than 75, (iii) diabetes, (iv) female gender, (v) hypertension, (vi) smoking, (vii) TIA,

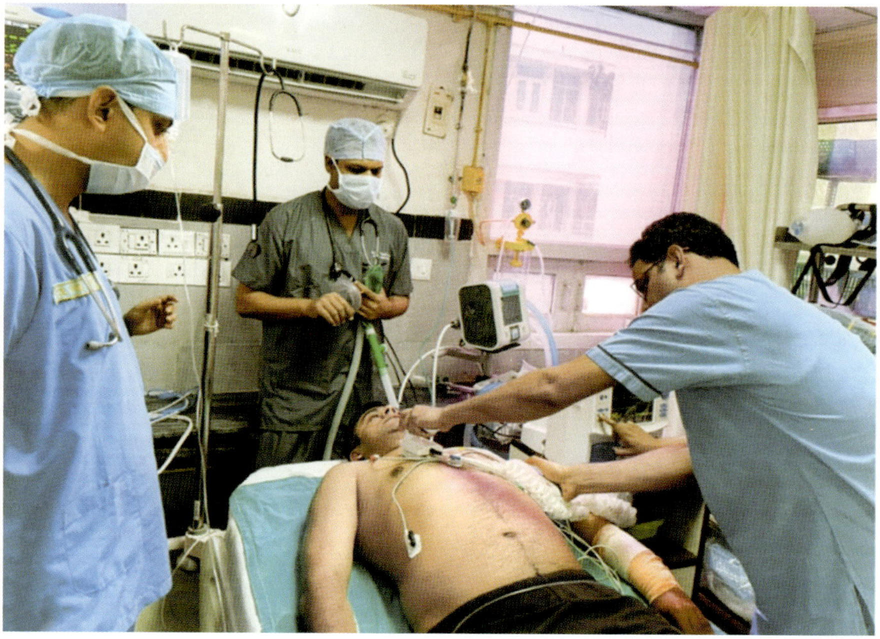

Fig. 5.25: DC conversion

or (viii) vascular disease. If score is up to 1 no anticoagulant is needed, if >2 then anticoagulant treatment with these agents can be given in the following doses:

i. **Dabigatran** 150 mg BD-thrombosis inhibitor
ii. Rivaroxaban factor Xa inhibitor 15–20 mg OD
iii. Apixaban Xa inhibitor 2.5 mg BD

} No prothrombin time estimation required

DC cardioversion (Fig. 5.25): Using 300 joules with synchronized R wave DC shock with facilities for endotracheal intubation or oximetry should be available in every district level hospital. Before DC conversion Midazolam 1–2 mg IV, even up to 5 mg should be given. It is urgently used in patients with fast heart rate, acute MI, LVF, low BP and also give IV heparin if Afib is less than 48 hours. No anticoagulants needed if Afib more than 48 hours. Preferably anticoagulant should be given for 3 weeks (elective case) and for 4 weeks after DC conversion. Oesophageal echocardiography to be done to exclude clot in LA in each case by a cardiologist very well trained in this procedure.

To summarize: Urgent termination of AF with injection **ibutilide**, or amiodarone, or metoprolol, or diltiazem.

DC cardioversion 300 joules followed by a maintenance dose of amiodarone, metoprolol, or dofetilide 0.25 mg OD or dronedarone 400 mg BD. Anticoagulant are with warfarin or clopidogrel with INR 2.5–3.1 in RHD case.

In other non-rheumatic cases new novel oral anticoagulants used. If facilities available catheter ablation after EPS studies to be done. Digoxin in CCF if it persists after AF conversion.

AV–Block P–R Interval (Fig. 5.26)

Distance measured from the beginning of P wave to the beginning of R wave. Normal P–R interval is 0.12 to 0.2 sec.

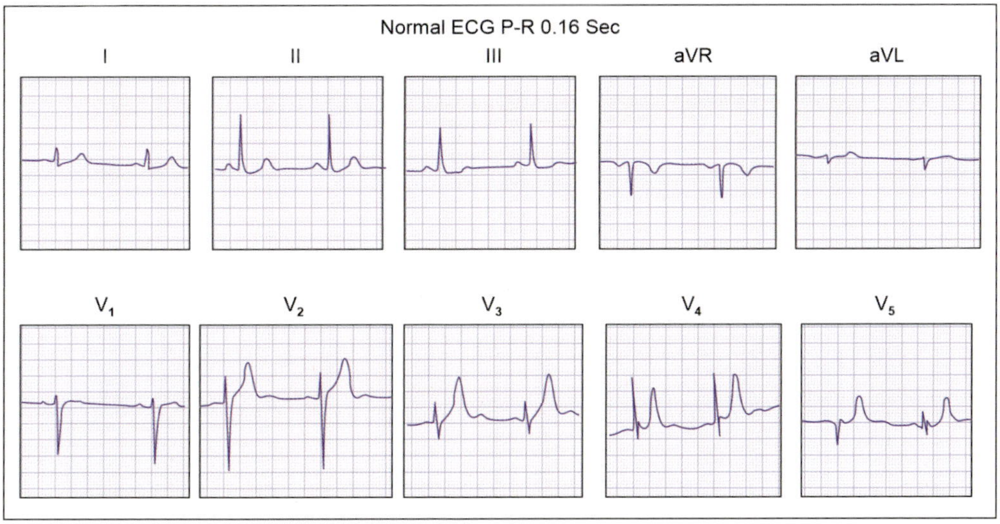

Fig. 5.26: Normal ECG P-R 0.16 sec

Short PR: <0.12 sec

Causes

1. Lown-Ganong-Levine (LGL) syndrome (Fig. 5.27).
2. Wolff-Parkinson-White (WPW) syndrome (in WPW syndrome the delta wave is seen in I, aVL, V_3 (Fig. 5.28).

Prolonged PR: >.20 sec 1st Degree AV Block

Causes

1. Congenital
2. IHD (Rt coronary artery disease) (Fig. 5.29)

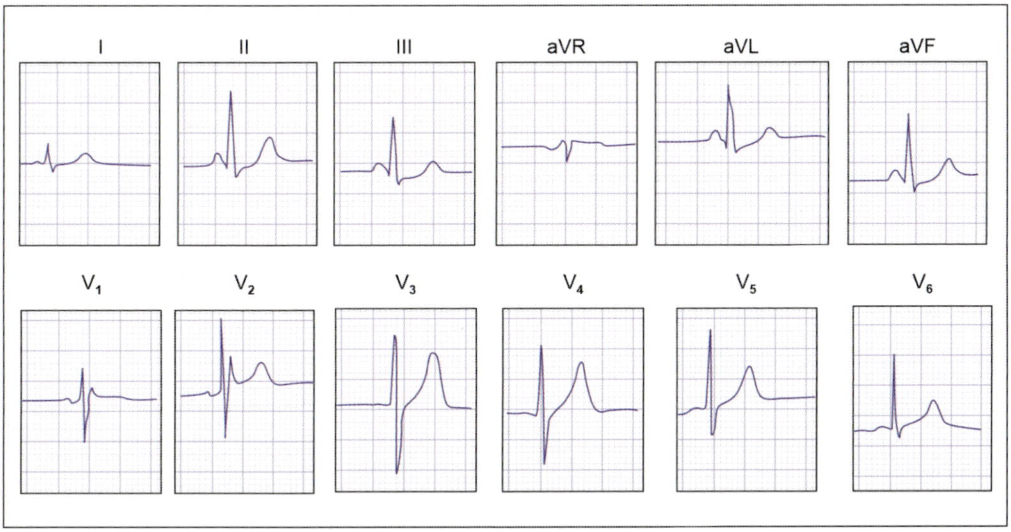

Fig. 5.27: LGL-short P-R interval P-R 0.1 sec

5

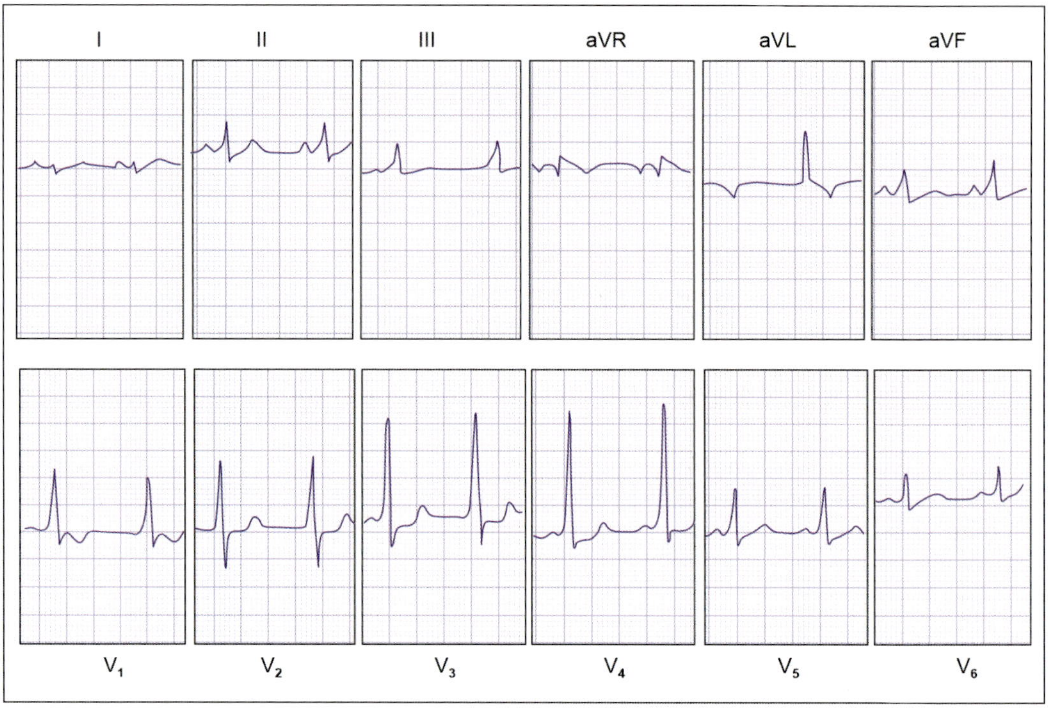

Fig. 5.28: WPW syndrome—Short P-R (0.08 Sec) and delta wave in V_2, V_3, V_4

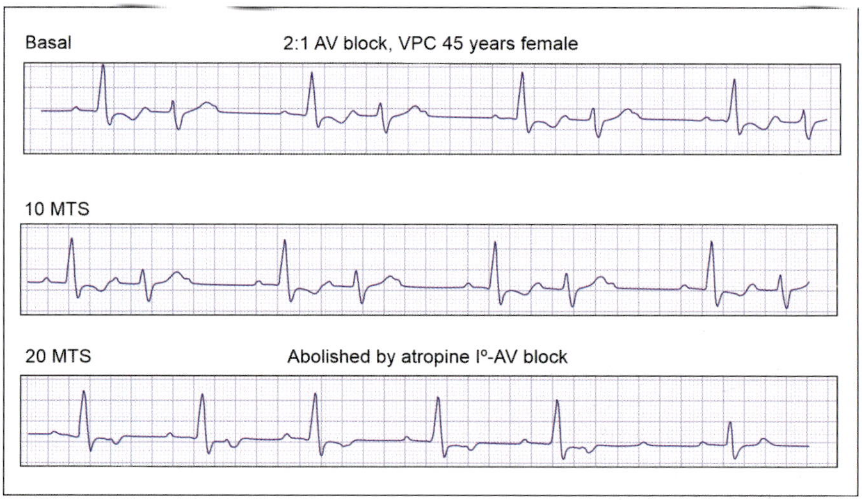

Fig. 5.29: 1°-AV block grade I P-R 0.32 Sec

3. Degeneration (Senile)
4. Increased vagal tone in athletes.

2nd Degree AV Block: 2 Types

5

a. When there is a progressive prolongation of P–R interval and after 3–4 cycles P wave drops and then there is no QRS complex. This is called **Wenckebach's phenomenon (Mobitz type 1)** (Fig. 5.30).

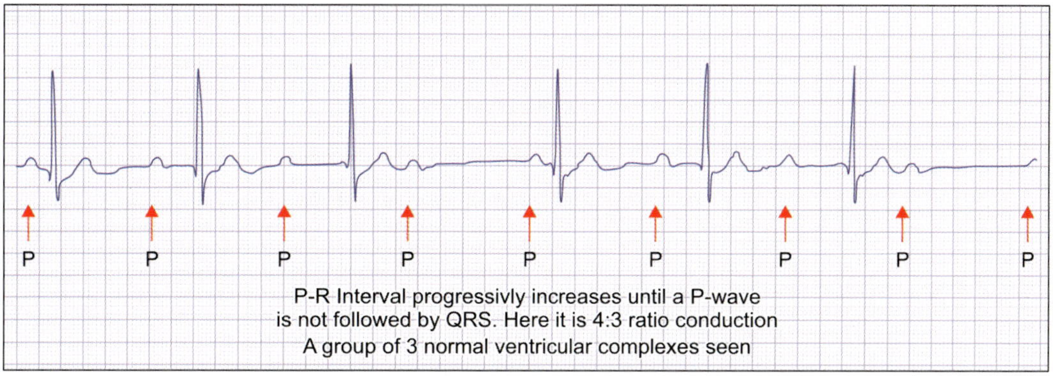

Fig. 5.30: 2nd degree AV block (Mobitz type-1) Wenckebach phenomenon

b. **Mobitz type 2:** Sudden dropping of P wave with normal rate. No QRS is seen after P wave. Sometimes, a regular 2:1 AV block is seen after 2 P waves. There is one QRS complex seen (Fig. 5.31).

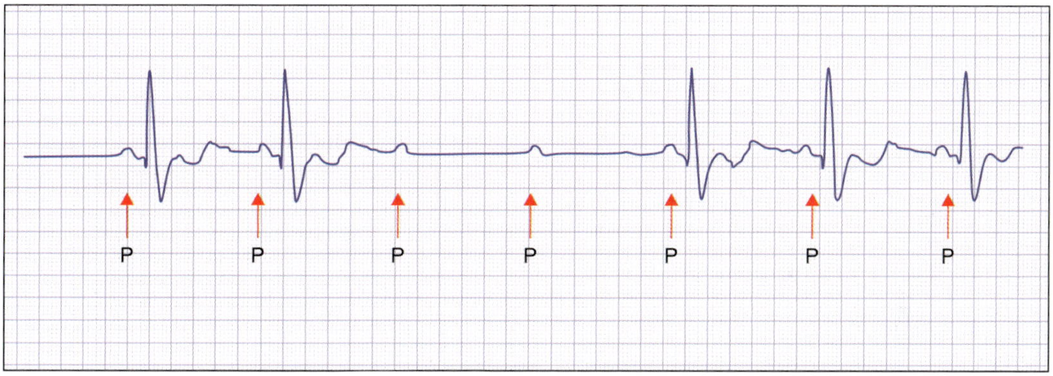

Fig. 5.31: Heart rate 25 per minute PR 0.22 seconds Mobitz type 2 AV block

3rd Degree AV Block

No AV conduction occurs and P–P intervals and QRS intervals are different. One may get narrow QRS in supra His block or mostly broad QRS is seen in ECG. They are discordant (Fig. 5.32). Heart rate is less than 40 and may get as low as 30 or 20 bpm. Patient gets syncope (Adams-Stokes).

Patient requires urgent hospital care and temporary cardiac treatment—pacemaker implantation followed by permanent dual chamber pacemaker implantation at the earliest.

Causes

1. Inferior wall MI
2. Drugs like digoxin, beta-blockers, calcium channel blockers
3. Idiopathic fibrosis of conduction tissue in AV node congenital defect
4. Aortic valve calcification
5. Postcardiac surgery trauma.

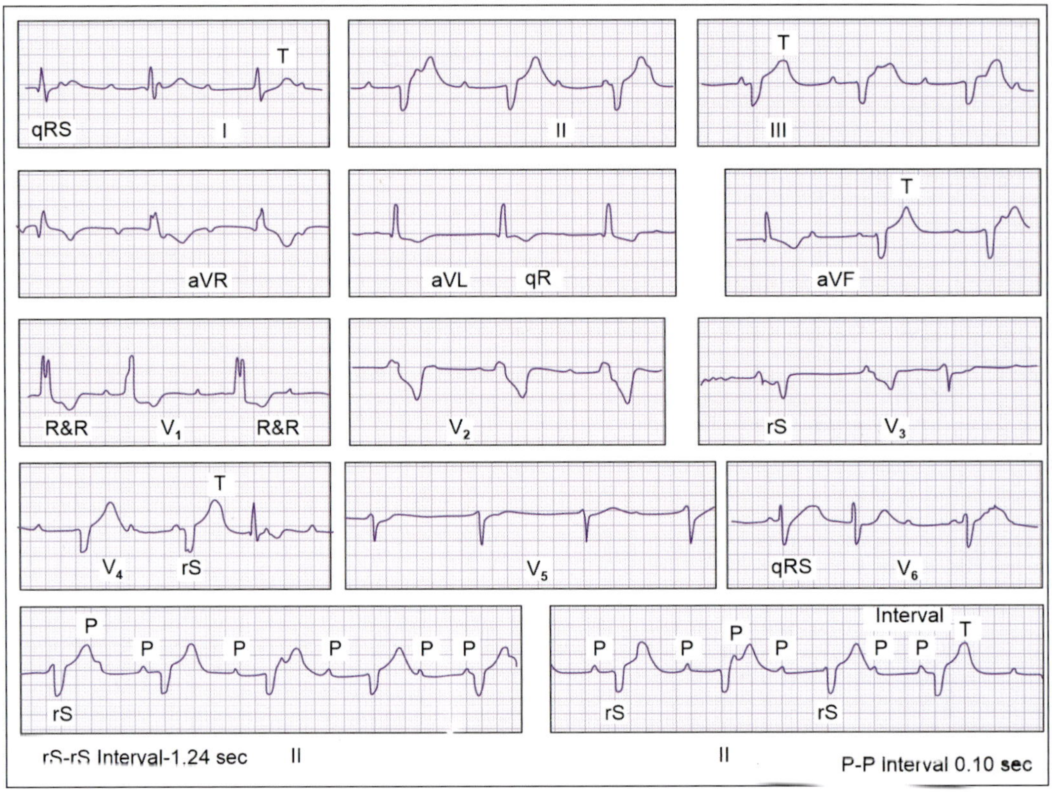

Fig. 5.32: Complete heart block

Variable PR Intervals

a. Wenckebach phenomenon
b. 3rd degree–AV block
c. Mobitz type II block.

Ventricular QRS Complex

i. AV block is broad, M or W shape as the focus is in ventricular muscle.
ii. Normal QRS duration is less than three small squares but in ventricular complexes QRS is broadened followed by an inverted T wave.

Intraventricular Conduction (IVC) Delay

When intraventricular conduction is less than 0.11 seconds but does not fulfil the criteria of left bundle branch block or right bundle branch block as enumerated below is called IVC delay.

Left Bundle Branch Block (LBBB)

When PR interval is normal but one of branches of His bundle is diseased and does not conduct cardiac impulses and so QRS complex is widened due to late depolarisation of areas of left ventricle after right ventricle is normally stimulated. It does not impair cardiac function.

LBBB Shows (Fig. 5.33)

- Loss of septal Q-wave seen in precordial limb leads.
- Widened, notched QRS complex in I, AVL, V_5, V_6 leads, S wave in lead AVF.
- QRS duration more than 0.12 seconds.
- Notched ascending R wave in leads I, AVL, V_5 and V_6.

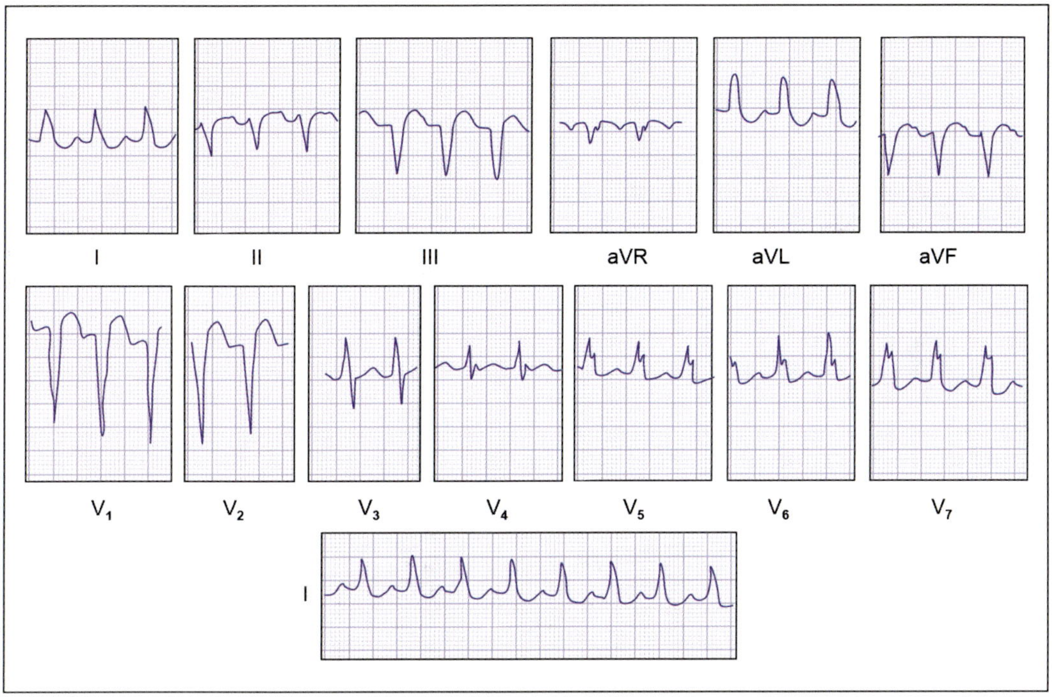

Fig. 5.33: Anteroseptal MI with LBBB 40 years female

Causes

1. Hypertension with LVH
2. Dilated cardiomyopathy
3. Ischaemic heart disease (anterior wall MI)
4. Commonly associated with organic heart disease
5. HOCM.

Right Bundle Branch Block (Figs 5.34 and 5.35)

- QRS > 0.12 seconds
- Secondary R′ wave in V_1, V_2 as rSR′ pattern
- Wide S wave in leads I, V_5, V_6 (more than 40 m/s).

Causes

1. Acute MI (Inf. wall mostly)
2. Acute pulmonary embolism
3. Chronic Cor pulmonale

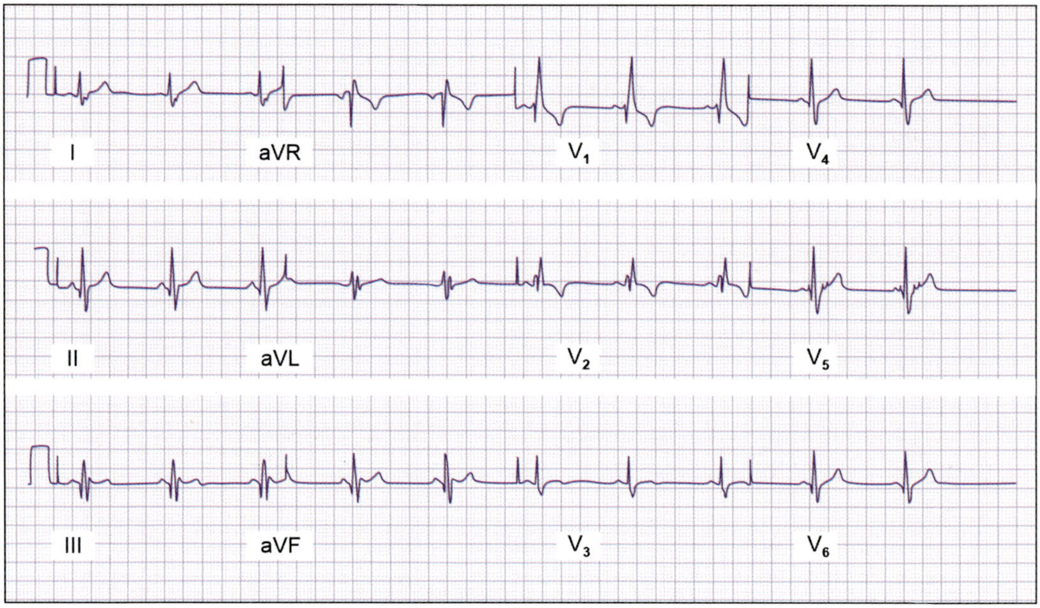

Fig. 5.34: 24 years man rSR pattern in V1
Classical RBBB = S wave in AVL, V_5, V_6, rSR in V_1

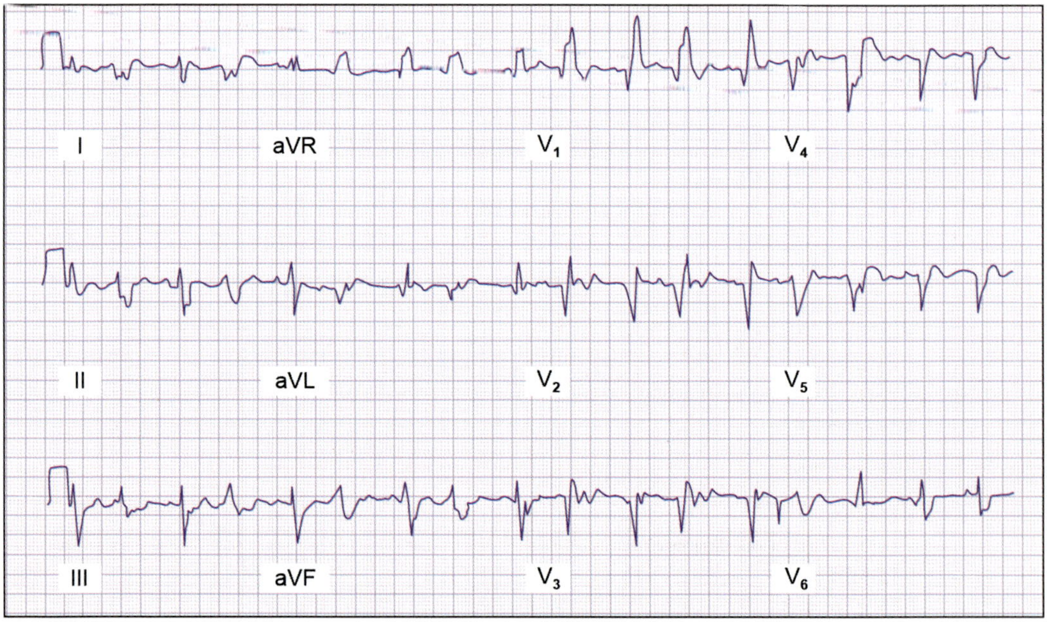

Fig. 5.35: Anteroseptal MI with QRBBB

5

4. ASD
5. Sometimes in healthy individuals, who have RBBB right from childhood and there is no evidence of organic heart disease.

Fascicular Blocks

When only one of two fascicles of left bundle is blocked

1. Left anterior fascicular block (LAFB): (Fig. 5.36)

   ECG shows

   i. Sinus rhythm
   ii. Normal PR interval
   iii. Left axis deviation
   iv. QRS duration less than 0.120 seconds
   v. RS in II, III, aVF
   vi. Q_1S_3

2. Left posterior fascicular block (LPFB) (Fig. 5.37)

   i. Axis more than 180°
   ii. RS in I, aVL, aVR, II, III, AVF
   iii. S_1Q_3.

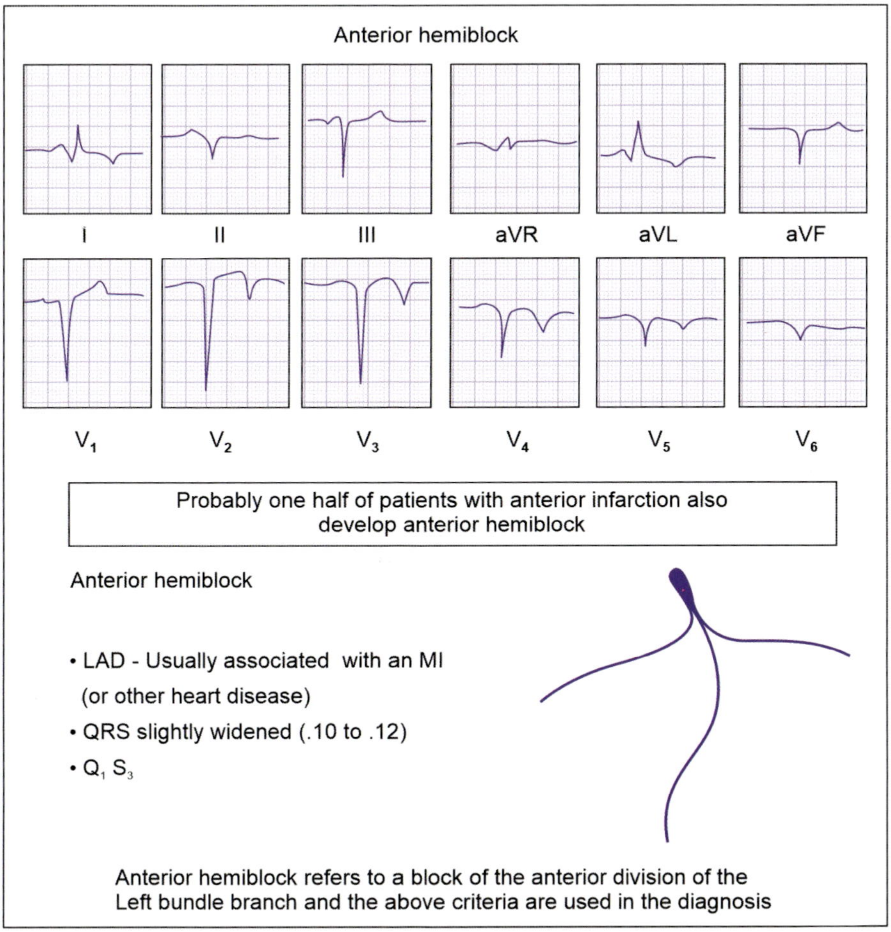

Fig. 5.36: Anterior hemiblock

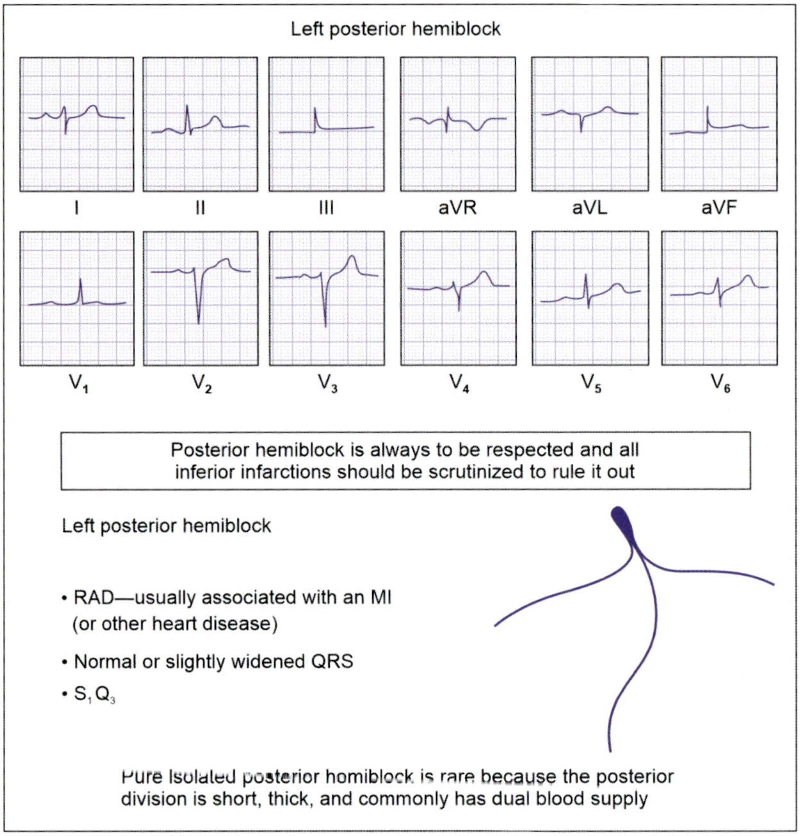

Fig. 5.37: Posterior hemiblock

CHAMBER ENLARGEMENT

1. Left Atrial Enlargement (Fig. 5.38)

Rheumatic heart disease (RHD) with severe **mitral stenosis with pulmonary hypertension** causes dilation of LA and is seen in ECG as **P mitrale** and **bifid P waves with terminal negativity >1 mm especially in V_1, II**. P wave duration is more than 120 m/s. P mitrale classically is seen in mitral stenosis. Dilated P wave, rarely is bifid pattern, is seen in LVH with raised LVEDP (left ventricular end-diastolic pressure) also in cases with severe MR due to any cause and accelerated hypertension.

2. Right Atrial Enlargement (Fig. 5.39)

P wave amplitude is > 0.25 milli volt in II, it is tall, more than 3 mm, and pointed seen in cases of acute Cor pulmonale as in pulmonary embolism and congestive heart failure in acute pulmonary embolism, sharp tell is seen.

3. Left Ventricular Enlargement (Fig. 5.40)

By Sokolow-Lyon criteria: S in V_1 + R in V_5 or V_6 > 35 mm, R in aVL >11 mm (Fig. 5.41).

5

Cornell voltage criteria: S in V_3 + R in aVL >28 mm in men and more than 20 mm in women.

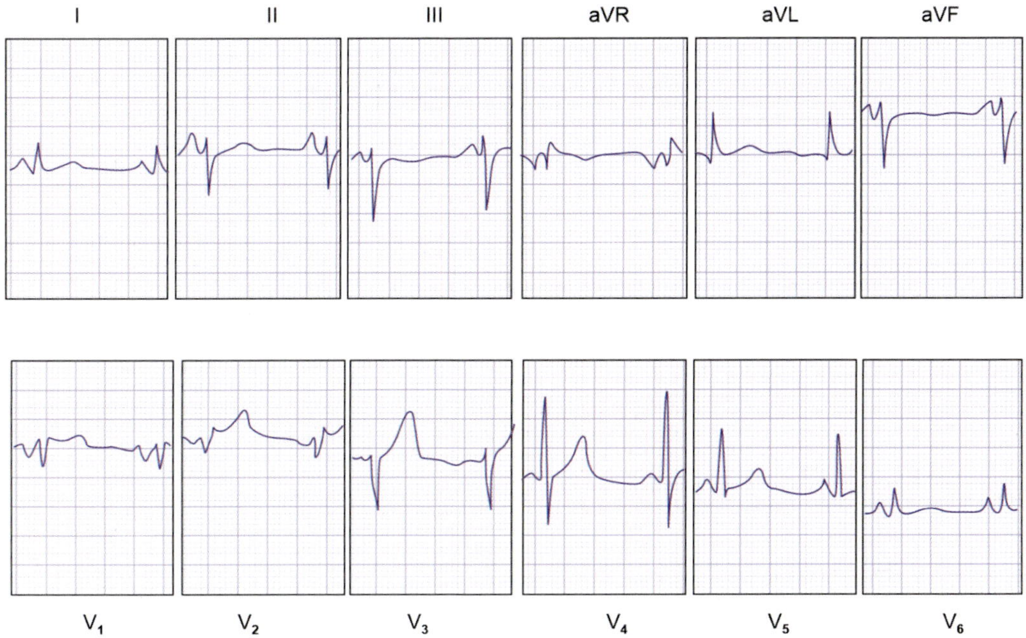

Left atrial enlarged and dilated
P Mitral negative mitral component of wave dilated, mitral stenosis

Fig. 5.38: Left atrial enlargement

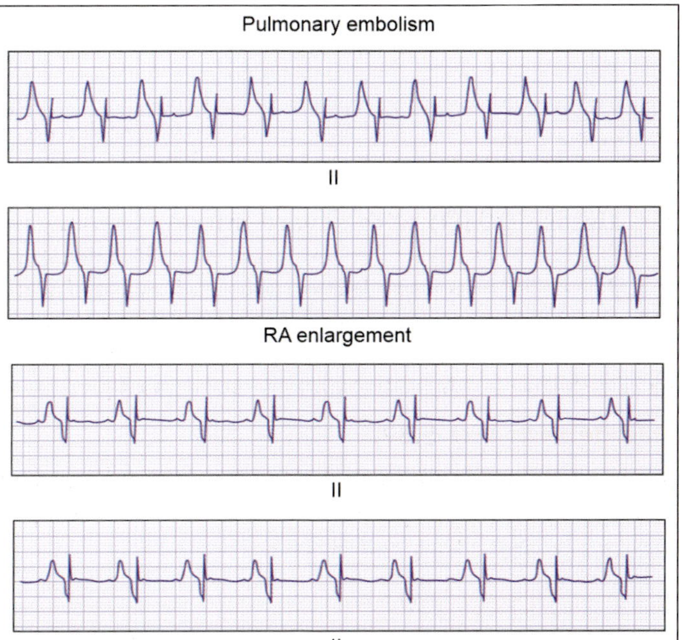

P–pulmonale
Sinus tachycardia–100 per minute

Fig. 5.39: Right atrial enlargement

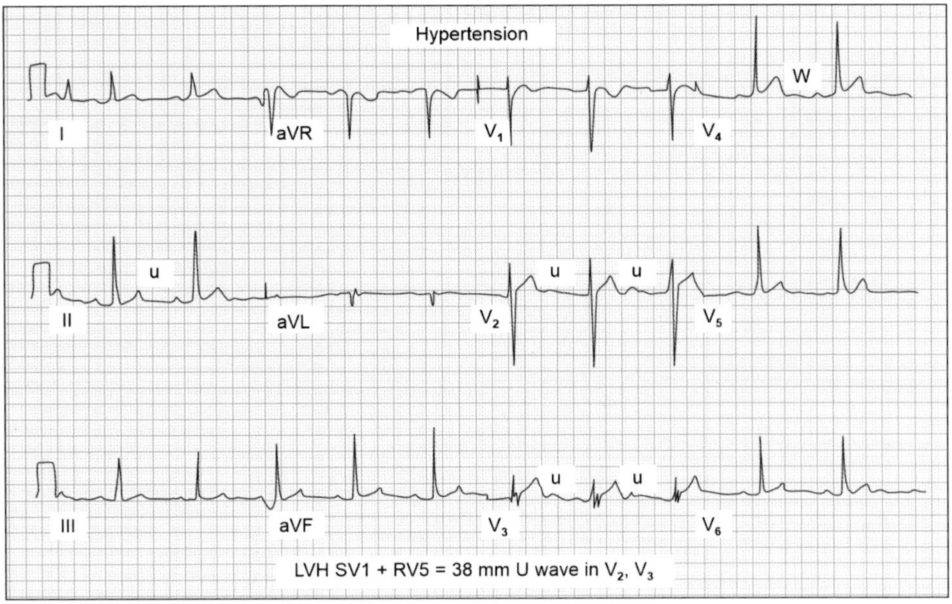

Fig. 5.40: LVH

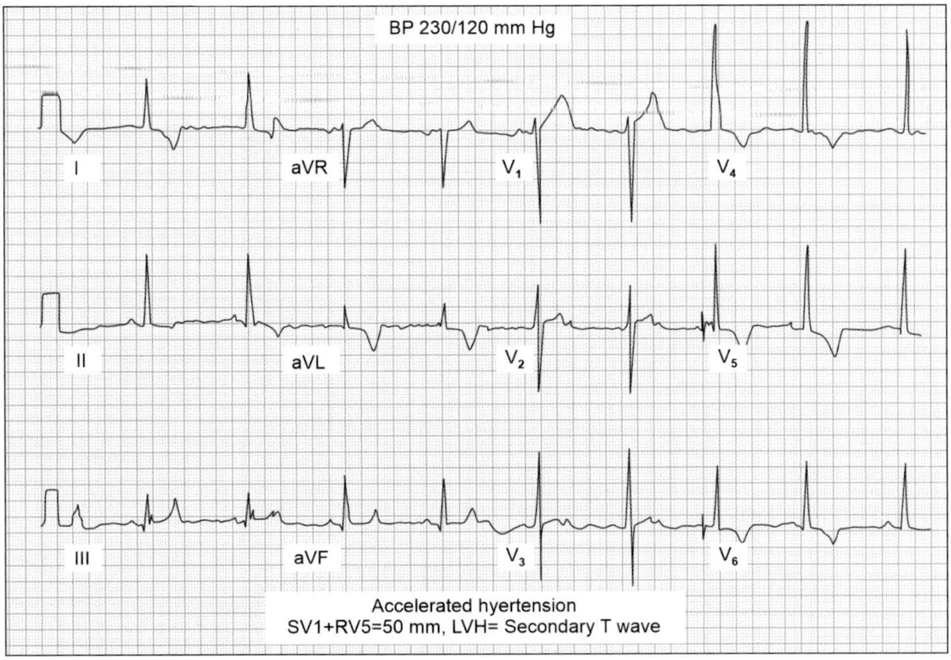

Fig. 5.41: Accelerated hypertension

Causes

1. Essential hypertension
2. Aortic stenosis
3. HOCM
4. Aortoarteritis.

4. Right Ventricular Hypertrophy (Fig. 5.42)

i. Tall R wave in V_1
ii. Right axis deviation
iii. QRS duration normal
iv. ST depression and T inversion in V_1, V_2
v. Prominent S wave in V_5, V_6.

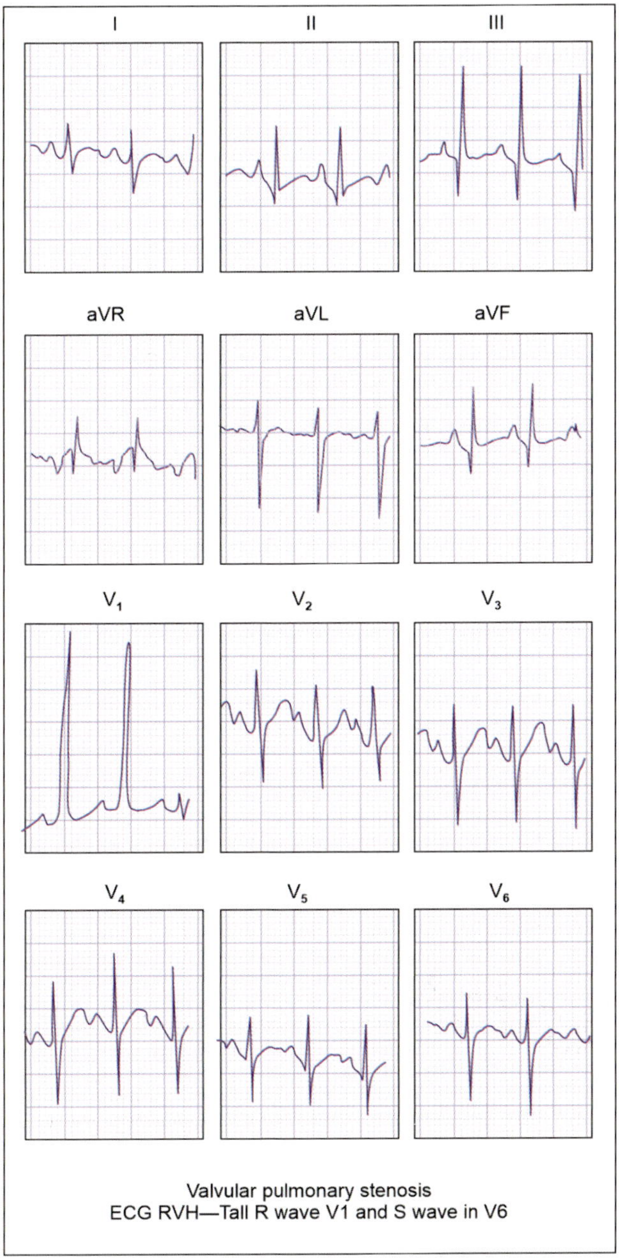

Fig. 5.42: Right ventricular hypertrophy

Causes

1. Mitral stenosis with PAH
2. Pulmonary stenosis
3. TOF (cyanotic heart disease)
4. TR.

Figure 5.43 shows both LVH and RVH morphological diagrams of the heart with deviation vectors.

Electrical axis of heart as influenced by left and right ventricular hypertrophy Arrows indicate major electrical vectors of ventricular depolarisation.
A. Left ventricular hypertrophy High voltage in limb leads (R I+S III ≥25mm) or precordial leads (SV1 + RV6 or SV2 + RV5 ≥35mm). Often, left atrial enlargement. ST-T abnormalities (strain pattern).
B. Right ventricular hypertrophy Tall R wave in lead V1 (R >5 mm). T wave inverted in V1. Right axis deviation. Associated right atrial enlargement.

LVH: Vector left axis deviation
RVH: Vector right axis deviation

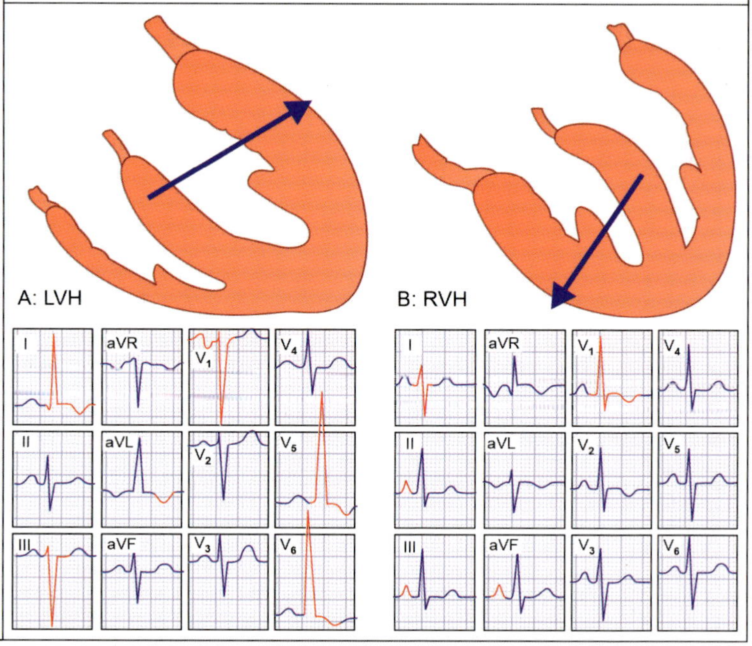

Fig. 5.43: Both RVH, LVH show morphological and ECG correlation

VENTRICULAR ARRHYTHMIAS

Three types of arrhythmias belong to this group of ECG disorders.

1. **Ventricular premature complexes (VPC)** or premature ventricular beat/complexes or regular premature depolarisation.
   All are synonyms or interchangeable
2. **Ventricular tachycardia**
3. **Ventricular flutter/fibrillation**
4. **Cardiac arrest**.

5

Ventricular Premature Contractions (Fig. 5.44)

These are premature ventricular depolarisation arising from right or left ventricle below the bundle of **His**.

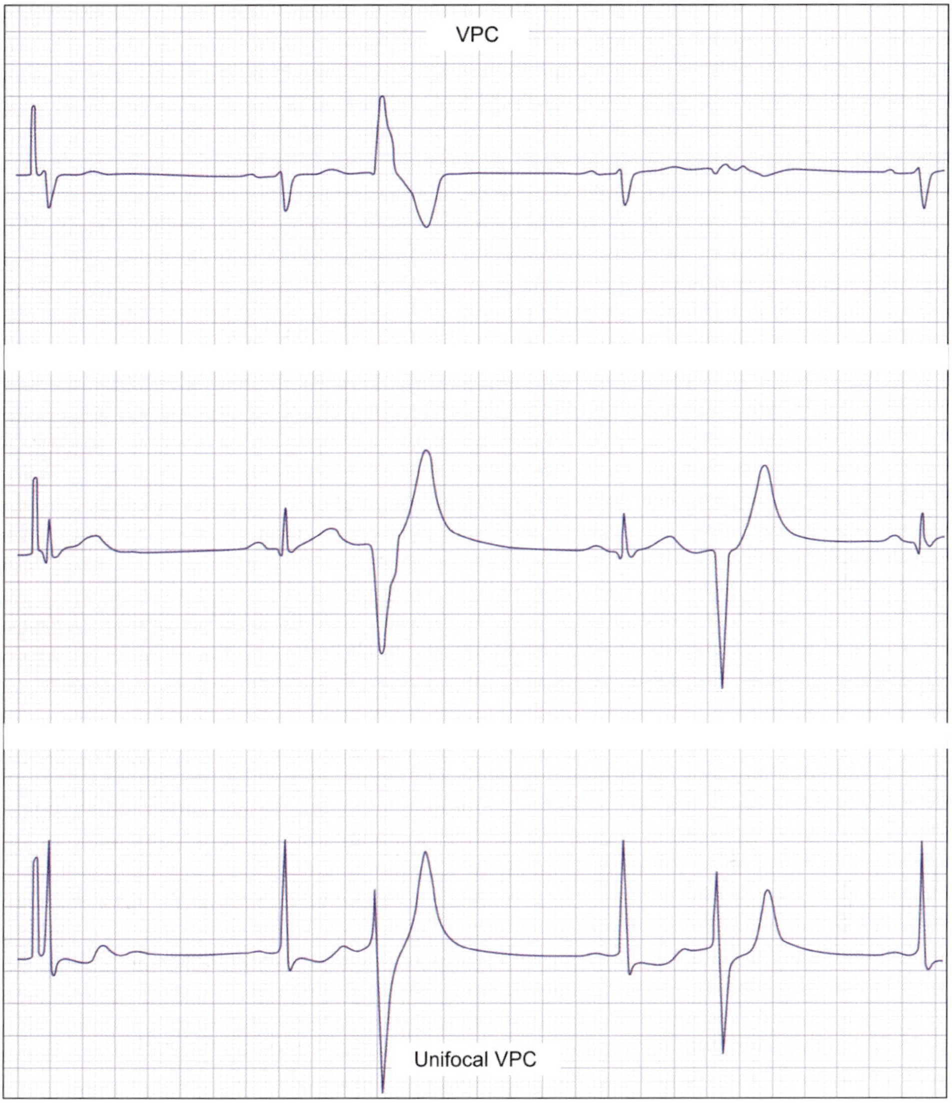

Fig. 5.44: Ventricular premature contractions

Characteristics of VPC (Figs 5.44 and 5.45)

- They are premature and occur earlier than normal expected beat, QRS complex is abnormal: Wide with W or M pattern of QRS.
- A broad wide >0.12 ms and QRS complex usually point to the opposite direction to sinus conducted beat. The impulse arises in the ventricular muscle and spreads to both ventricles slowly, hence it is wide and aberrant.
- RR interval is irregular.
- Sinus P wave appears just after QRS or is buried in it. VPC appears before sinus P wave. Sometimes P wave after VPC (QRS) appears inverted in shape as atrial depolarisation occurs from AV node to SA node by VPC impulse. P wave has never been seen before QRS complex in VPC.

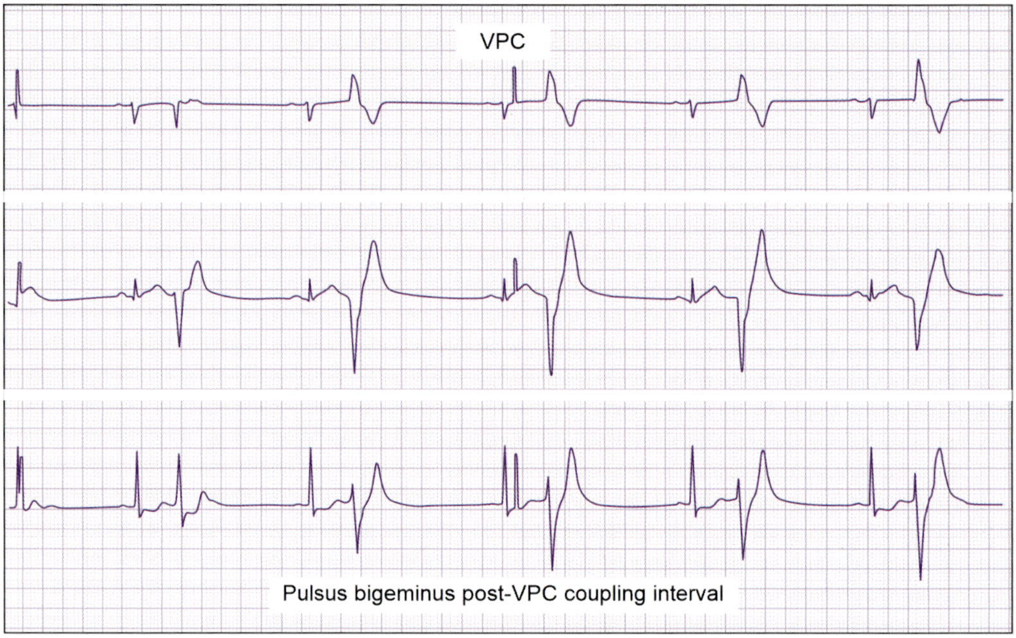

Fig. 5.45: Ventricular premature contractions

- **Compensatory pause:** The long time interval between ectopic QRS and normally conducted QRS is a compensatory pause. It is time taken by ventricle and atria to be repolarised after an ectopic beat. Sinus rhythm is retained. The distance between two normally conducted sinus beats that surround VPC is double the normal RR interval. VPC in some patients in different leads have different shapes.

Variants of VPC

1. VPC emerging in RV have LBBB pattern since LV is stimulated after the RV and ectopic starting in LV has RBBB pattern.
2. **Fusion beat (Dressler beat)** (Fig. 5.46)**:** VPC occurs at the same time as that of normal sinus impulse reaching the ventricle. P wave proceeding ectopic QRS comes on time, relevant QRS complex is a blend of partially normal depolarisation and partially abnormal depolarisation, hence fusion beat which is wider than normal narrower than VPC.
3. **Coupling interval:** Interval between VPC and normal preceding QRS complex is called coupling interval.
    1. VPC occurs alternatively with normal QRS–Bigeminy
    2. VPC occurs after two sinus beats trigeminy
    3. VPC occurs after three sinus beats quadrigeminy.
4. **Uniform VPC:** VPCs in one lead are identical in shape and come from one focus.
5. **Multiform or multifocal VPC:** VPC have different shapes in the same lead is easily identified as they are from multiple sites mostly organic and significant cardiac diseases, e.g. after post-MI.
6. **R-on-T phenomenon** (Fig. 5.47): VPC/VPB are so timed that they occur at the peak of the T wave of preceding normal sinus conducted beat. These VPCs usually precipitate

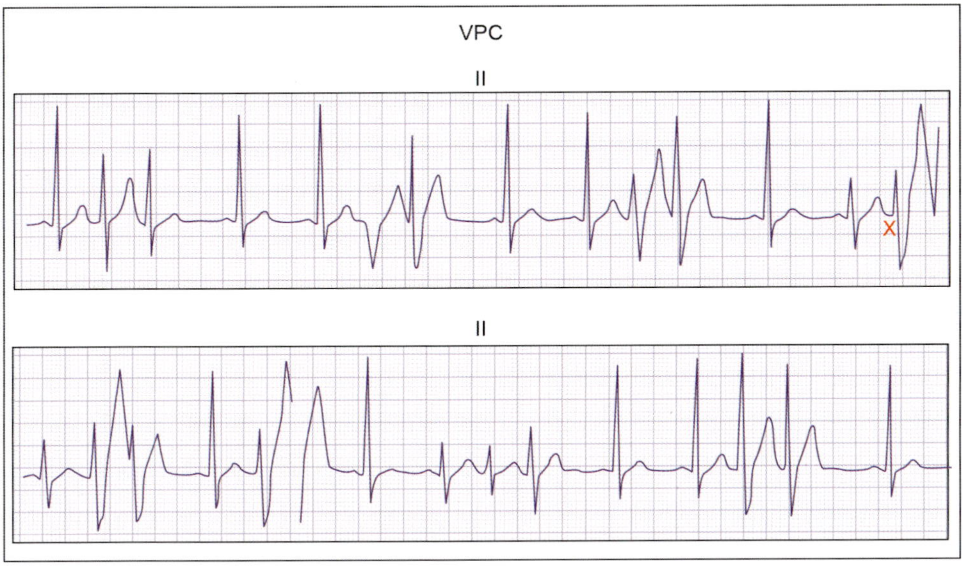

Fig. 5.46: VPC couplets few fusion beats seen (X)

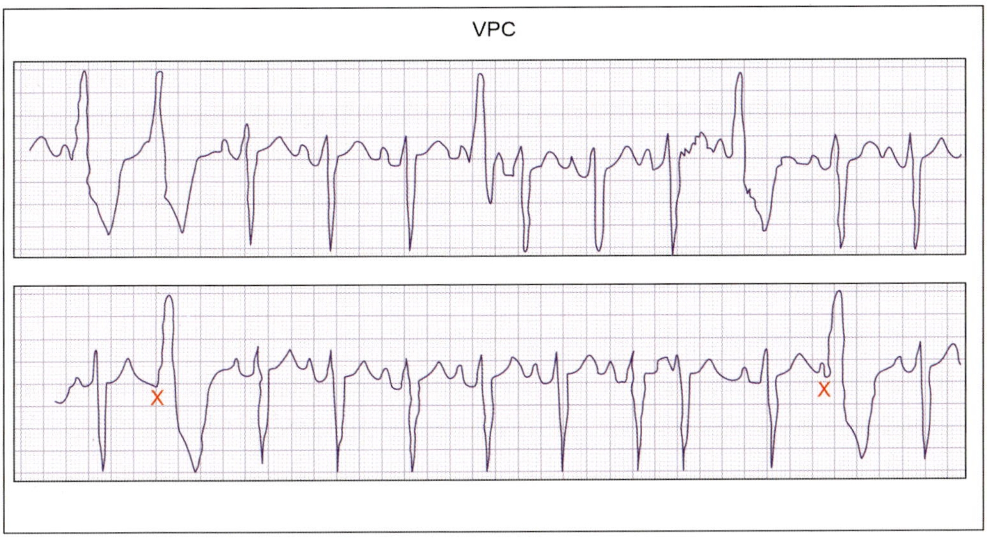

Fig. 5.47: VPC salvos and R-on-T phenomenon (X)

an episode of VT or VF in the course of AWMI (anterior wall myocardial infarction) or myocardial ischaemia and they cause long QT intervals.

7. Couplet 2 VPC is usually focal and multifocal in a row in the same lead.
8. Triplet three VPC together in a row termed VT.

Aetiology of VPC

1. It can be a normal finding if in Holter ECG monitor up to 8 VPCs are seen in 1000 beats, particularly in young adolescents and few people up to 30 years. There is no clinical evidence of heart disease (i.e. no cardiac murmur). ECG, X-ray, 2D echo

and Doppler study is normal and in some stress echocardiogram is normal. No biochemical abnormality was seen. We follow them every year for five years.
2. Benign cardiac lesion: **Mitral valve prolapse**, mild hypertension, innocent cardiac murmur.
3. Anxiety, diet pattern (fatty food no exercise), obesity
4. Diabetes mellitus
5. Essential hypertension
6. Heart disease
   a. Congenital heart disease
   b. Any cardiac surgery in childhood ASD, VSD, PDA
   c. RHD with valve involvement
   d. IHD in all forms (after CABG), cardiomyopathies of all types, post-reperfusion therapy in acute MI, acute medical emergency with low potassium, low magnesium, shock, decreased atmospheric oxygen (high altitude >10,000 ft), and hypothermia.
   e. COPD, post-pneumonia
   f. Pericarditis
   g. Old athletes.
   h. Post corona-19 infection.

Management

- A good history should be taken of all drugs, habit forming, dietary items excess, caffeine, alcohol or psychotropic drugs and opioids preparation, heroin derivatives, and smoking history. Use of aminophylline-based drugs and bronchodilator use.
- Clinical examination: To rule out hypertension, diabetes mellitus, COPD and CCF and to exclude organic heart disease as mentioned earlier.
- History of cardiac surgery.
- ECG, stress ECG, 24-hour Holter ECG, biochemistry, thyroid profile to exclude thyrotoxicosis, echocardiography, stress, echo, X-ray heart.
- CT chest if needed and MRI heart to be done if signs of congenital heart disease or cardiomyopathy are suspected.
- History of cardiac drugs like digoxin, quinidine, and drugs that prolong QT interval.
- After total evaluation and good discussion with patient and his/her parents the drug treatment may be initiated, in VPC, especially with **fusion beat, triplets, R-on-T phenomenon**, the aim is to prevent cardiac arrest, ventricular fibrillation, and ventricular tachycardia.

For those without structural heart disease with symptoms of palpitations or syncope and multifocal VPC, R-on-T phenomenon and exercise-induced VPC. It is recommended:

1. Beta-adrenergic drugs: Metoprolol 25 mg BD or Sotalol or Carvedilol (especially in cases of IHD or cardiomyopathies).
2. Periodic check-up 1–2 months to exclude bradycardia or prolonged P-R interval or QT prolongation on ECG.

5

Ventricular Tachycardia (Fig. 5.48)

Definition: Rapid ventricular dysrhythmia due to run off three or more consecutive VPB occurring in the same ECG leads is ventricular tachycardia. QRS duration >100 milliseconds.

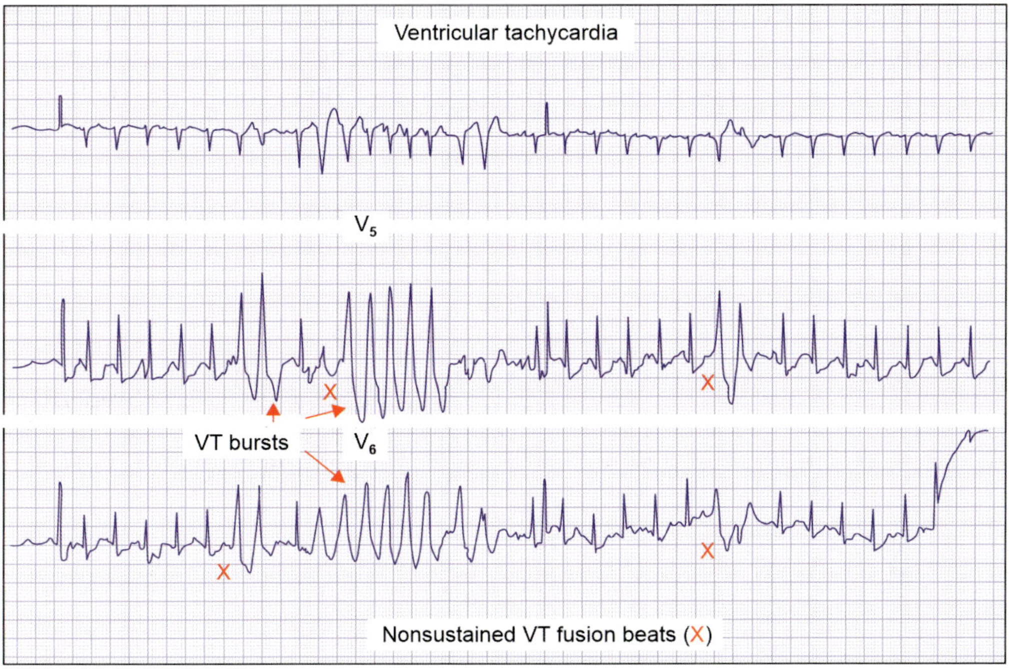

Fig. 5.48: Ventricular tachycardia

Classification

i. Non-sustained lasting less than 30 seconds or up to 3 beats (Fig. 5.48).
ii. Sustained lasting more than 30 seconds and associated with symptoms of giddiness, syncope or near syncope and hypotension.

Morphological Classification

i. **Monomorphic:** Same shape as QRS
ii. Polymorphic variable shape of QRS is seen in the same leads, in cases with long QT syndrome of IHD.
iii. **Concordant:** When the direction of QRS is same in all the precordial leads either positive or negative.
Discordant: Variable direction of broad QRS complexes in precordial leads.

Features Suggestive of VT

i. QRS duration >0.14 sec
ii. LAD –90 to –180 or NW (northwest) axis
iii. AV dissociation
iv. Fusion beats
v. Sustained VT with fusion beats (Fig. 5.49).

Patients with VT are usually very ill, admitted in ICU or ICCU. For OPD cases with history of syncope, very fast heart rate, giddiness, hypotension, ECG showing possibly

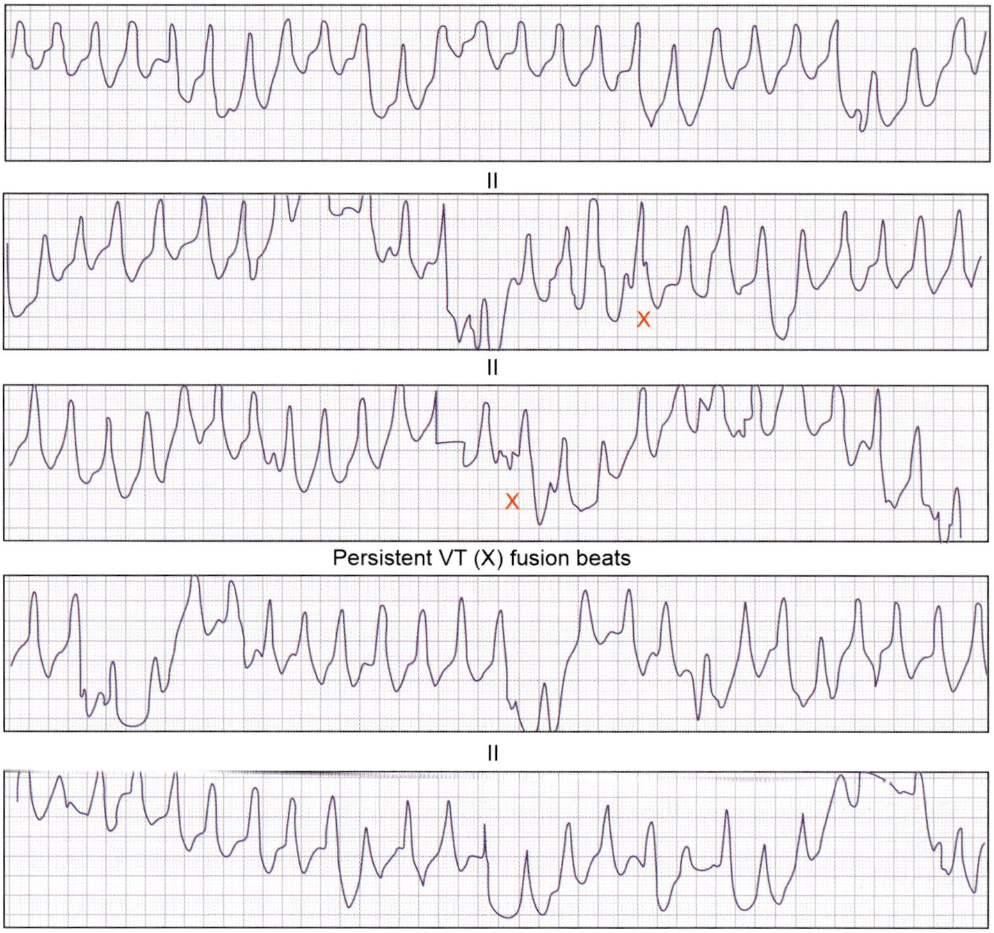

Fig. 5.49: Persistent VT fusion beats

VT, immediate attendance by residents and senior residents is required with urgent message to the consultants (medicine/cardiology) be given and these patient should be sent as fast as possible to ICU/ICCU for urgent treatment. These patients can go to sudden cardiac death as most of them have fairly advanced structural heart disease.

ECG Features of VT

i. QRS complex, wider more than 100 milliseconds are called wide QRS tachycardia
ii. All QRS complexes look alike
iii. Heart rate over 100 per minute and RR interval regular
iv. Ventricular fusion beat, Dressler's beat or sinus capture beats are seen
v. QRS complex in chest lead V_1 through V_6 are either positive or negative in VT.

VT/SVT with Aberration

This is a serious differential diagnosis of broad QRS tachycardia.

In Fig. 5.50, the ECG features of both of these ECG disorders are shown in V_1.

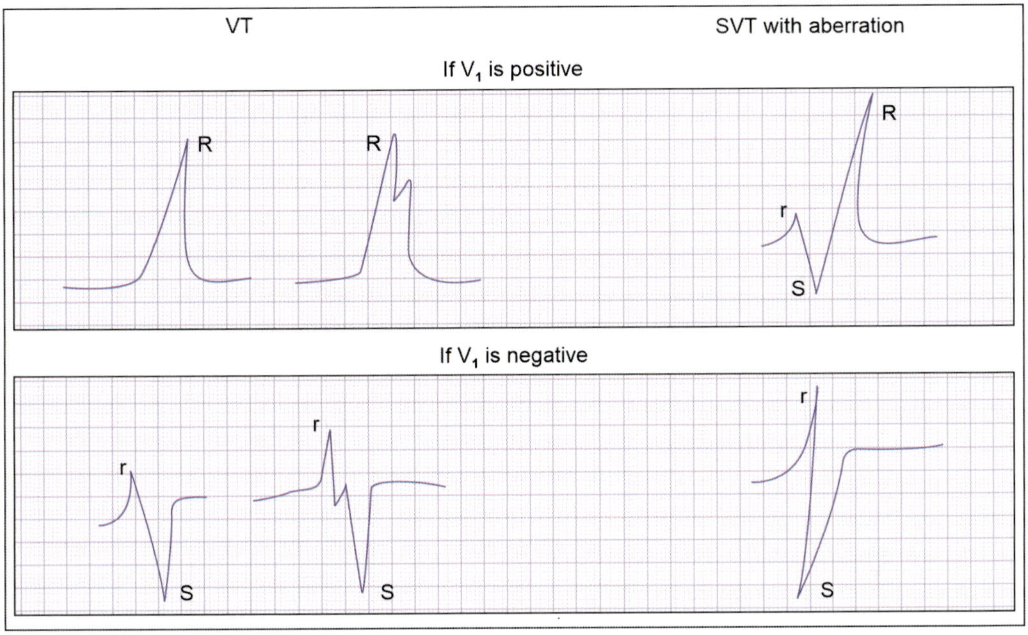

Fig. 5.50: VT/SVT with aberration

Causes of VT

1. Acute coronary syndrome (unstable angina/subendocardial MI)
2. Acute myocardial infarction
3. Acute myocarditis
4. Hypokalaemia
5. Hypomagnesaemia
6. Drugs like digoxin or other proantiarrhymic drugs
7. Mechanical stimulation of endocardium during pacing catheter insertion.
   i. Reperfusion after thrombolytic treatment of acute MI.
   ii. During cardiac surgery.

Treatment of VT

Cardioversion (Fig. 5.25)

This is the first line of treatment in cases of VT. **Facilities of endotracheal intubation with oxygen supply and oximetry should be stand by in the same room.** IV cannula to be inserted immediately **by a trained senior nursing staff**. 100 joules of synchronised R wave DC shock should be given after gel is applied on the precordium (over the midsternal area and the LV apical region patient on oxygen and slightly sedated with midazolam. If no improvement then repeat DC shock up to 300 joules.

Medical Treatment

Injection lignocaine IV 75 to 200 mg bolus given then 2 to 4 mg per min IV given for 24 to 30 hours.

5

Injection amiodarone IV 150 mg bolus in 10 minutes followed by 300 mg IV infusion in 6 hours then 540 mg infusion in remaining 24 hours. Later on oral dose of 200 mg daily is given.

After the acute phase the following investigations are to be done:

- Complete blood count
- LFT, RFT
- Thyroid profile
- Chest X-ray for cardiac size. If pacemaker is implanted, to be analysed for its functioning, by the local agent of the pacemakers supplying company as malfunctioning by a pacemaker can cause VT
- Coronary angiography
- Electrophysiological Study for detection of ectopic foci in the ventricles
- 24 hours Holter ECG monitoring
- 2 D echocardiography.

After discharge: Maintenance therapy by amiodarone or tab sotalol is advised.

Torsades de Pointes (Fig. 5.51)

(Polymorphic Ventricular Tachycardia)

In this type of VT, QRS direction rotates on its axis cyclically pointing downwards for several beats and then twisting and pointing upwards in the same lead.

Mechanism: Delayed ventricular depolarisation leads to prolonged QT interval. VPC with R and T phenomenon occurs, causing VT of this type. It is caused by a lot of commonly used cardiac drugs, like disopyramide, ibutulide, and amiodarone.

Predisposing factors: Hypokalaemia, long QT syndrome, temporary pacing.

Treatment: I/V magnesium sulphate (dose 1–2 gm IV slowly as it may cause hypotension) and DC cardioversion.

Ventricular Flutter (Fig. 5.52)

Rapid ventricular tachycardia with a rate of 250 to 300 per minute. It is a precursor of ventricular fibrillation.

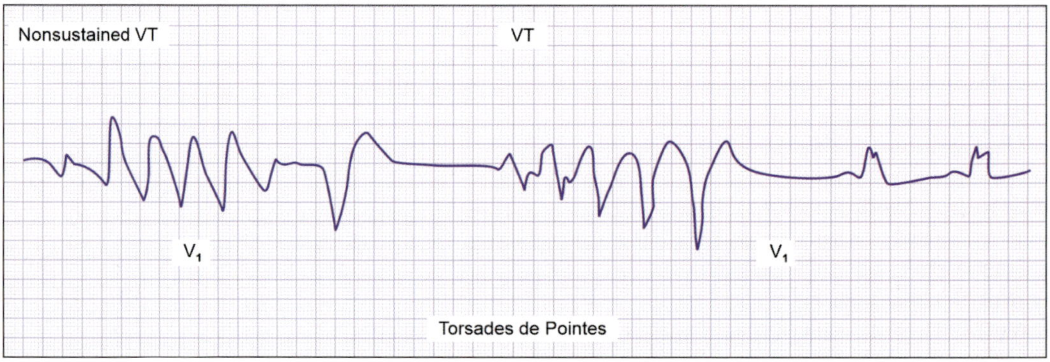

Fig. 5.51: Torsades de pointes

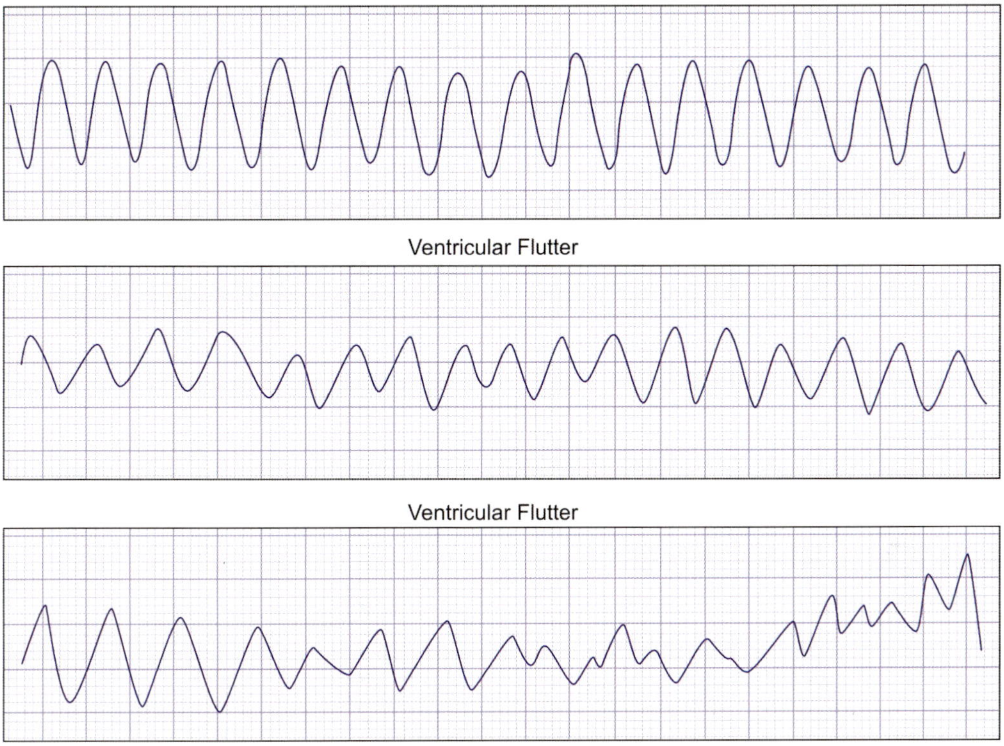

Fig. 5.52: Ventricular flutter

ECG: QRS complex as well as ST and T waves are difficult to make out due to large amplitude T waves which appear continuously with no baseline visible. Causes the same as VT.

Treatment: Rapid and urgent as previously detailed for VT (ventricular tachycardia) haemodynamic collapse can occur any time when ventricular flutter can degenerate to ventricular fibrillation and then cardiac arrest.

Rapid cardioversion from 100 to 300 joules.

Drugs as in VT. Injection lignocaine, amiodarone useful

Repeat cardioversion

Life support CPR. To be kept ready.

Ventricular Fibrillation (Fig. 5.53)

Catastrophic dysrhythmia due to total disintegration of cardiac electrical activity. ECG monitor shows no ECG wave form but underlying wavy baseline fibrillatory wave varying in amplitude and morphology after some time fibrillatory waves become smaller than VT waves. This fine VF can go to stand still and ECG shows a straight line

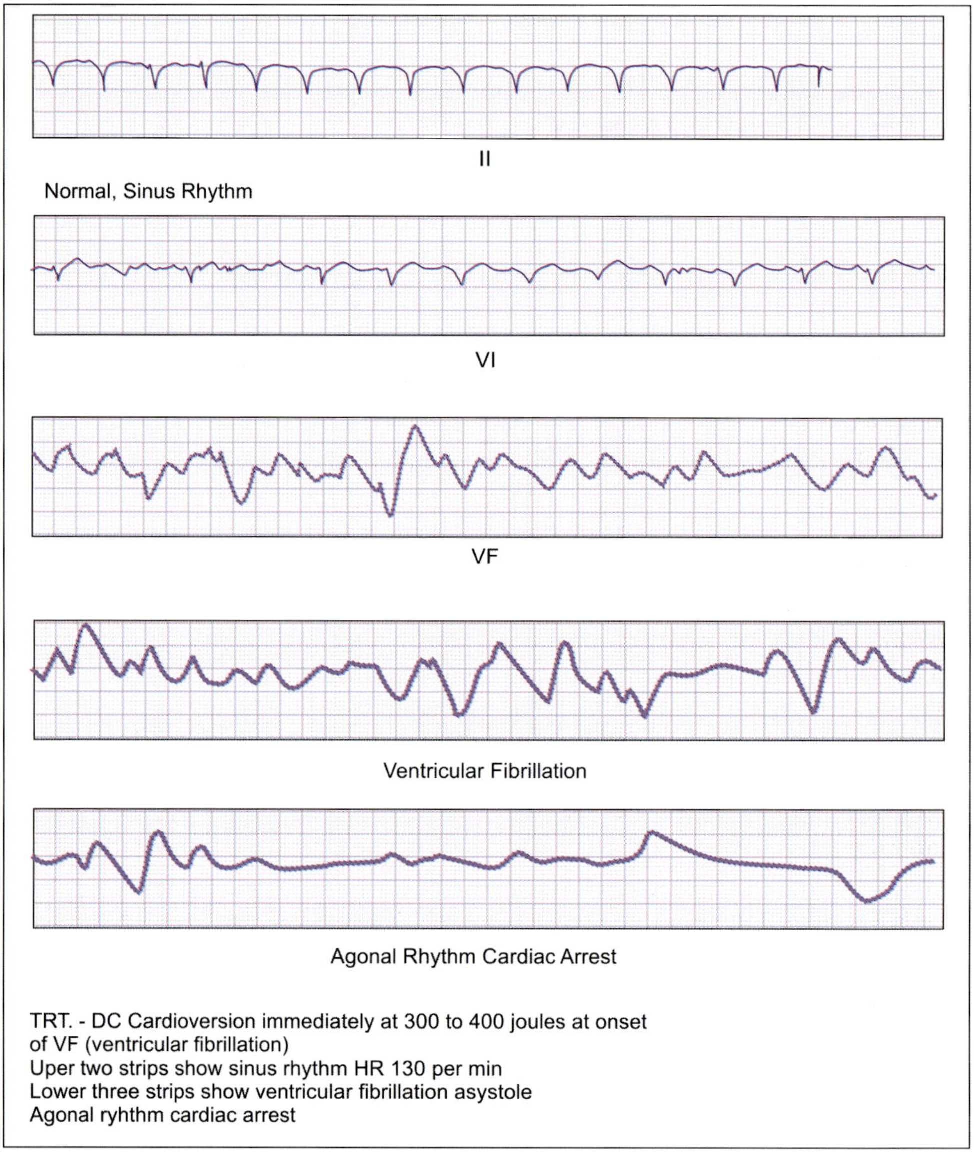

Fig. 5.53: Ventricular fibrillation

with an agonal rhythm. Continue CPR for 6 hr as is common hospital policy. Declare dead after consulting, Senior anaesthetiest/senior physician/senior cardiologist. CPR protocol is discussed in subsequent pages treatment of cardiac arrest.

Chapter 6

ECG Changes in Ischaemic Heart Disease

CORONARY CIRCULATION (Fig. 6.1a and b)

Basically, there are **two coronary arteries right and left**, coming out of proximal part of ascending aorta, just above the aortic valve. Right from right coronary sinus and left from left coronary sinus.

Left main coronary artery (LCA) or left main stem: It traverses maximally up to 2.5 cm and then divides into two branches.

1. **Left anterior descending (LAD) artery:** It runs in anterior interventricular groove down to LV inferior border.
2. **Left circumflex artery (LCX):** It runs posteriorly in atrioventricular groove.

LAD gives branches to supply the anterior part of septum (septal perforator septal 1 and septal 2) and to anterior and lateral wall branches (1st diagonal and 2nd diagonal branches to supply arterial blood to anterior, lateral and apical wall of LV (left ventrical).

LCX gives marginal branches (OMI and OM_2) that supply blood to posterior, inferior and lateral wall of LV.

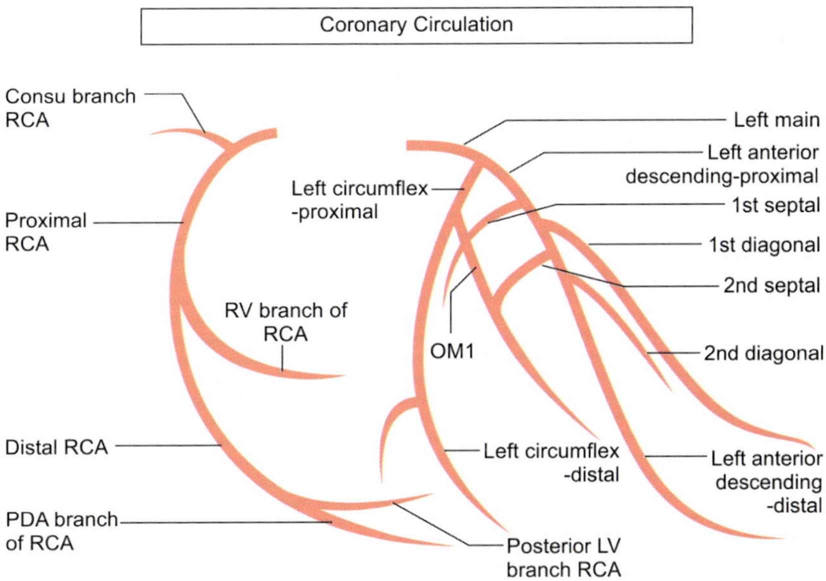

LV, left ventricle; PDA, posterior descending artery; RCA, right coronary artery

Fig. 6.1a: The schematic diagram of some branches of coronary arteries

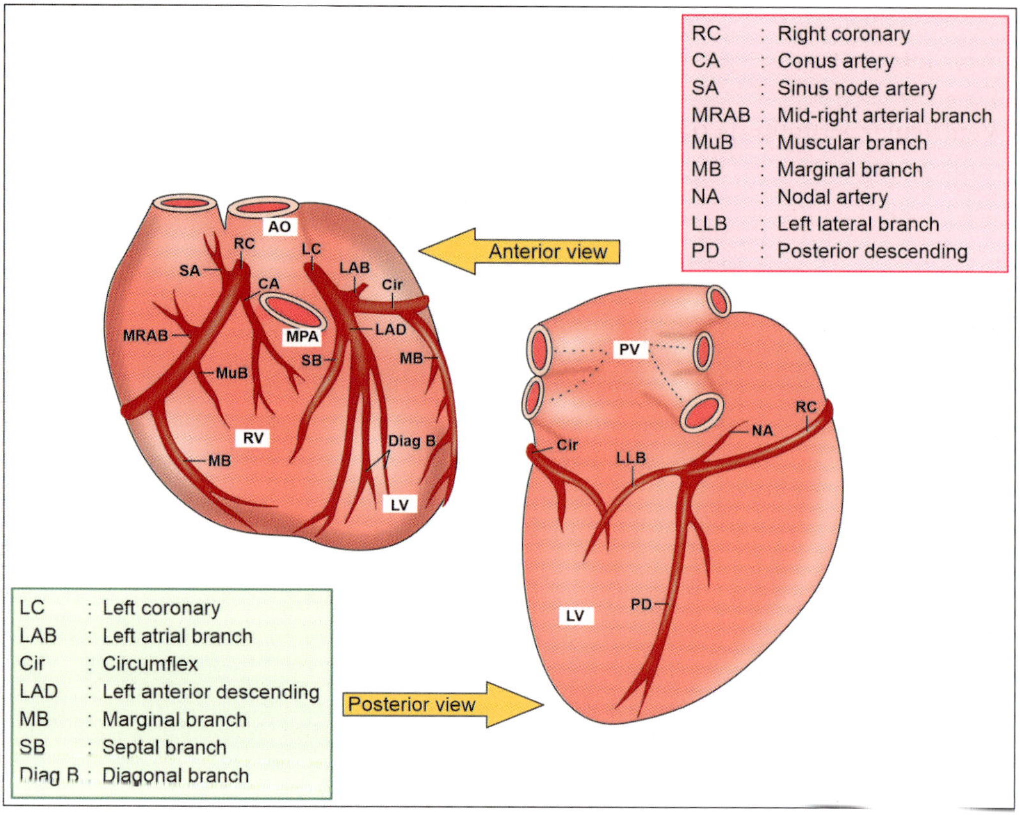

Fig. 6.1b: Coronary circulation

Right coronary artery (RCA): It runs in right atrioventricular groove, giving branches to supply arterial blood to **SA node, AV node, RA, RV and infero-posterior segment of LV, PDA** (posterior descending artery) branch of distal RCA, runs in post-interventricular groove and supplies inferior part of IV. Septum in 90% of cases who have **dominant RCA system of coronary circulation**. In remaining 10% it is supplied by the **LCX branch**.

RCA supplies SA node in 60% cases and AV node in 90% cases through its nodal artery branch. So in proximal occlusion of RCA sinus bradycardia occurs abrupt RCA closure causes inferior (LV) MI/RV infarction.

ECG Changes in IHD (Ischaemic Heart Disease)

IHD, due to coronary atherosclerosis is very common in India and South Asia with a prevalence of 14% in the urban population and 7.8% in the rural areas, based on seven-fold increase in urban cases and 4.5 fold increase in rural areas, in the last 50 years in India. It appears to be an underestimate.

IHD Presents as the Following Clinical Syndromes

1. Stable: Angina pectoris
2. Unstable: Angina
3. ST elevated: Acute myocardial infarction
4. Non-ST elevated: Acute myocardial infarction

(Items 2–4: } Acute coronary syndrome)

5. Asymptomatic microvascular angina
6. Cardiomyopathy
7. Ventricular arrhythmia (Discussed in detail in Chapter 5)
8. Sudden death

Stable Angina Pectoris

For diagnoses of angina pectoris besides clinical signs and symptoms of chest pain, an ECG examination is essential.

The ECG changes in angina pectoris will be discussed as per the latest classification of IHD which is accepted at present as indicated in the above paras.

ECG Changes in Stable Effort Angina

1. **Classical ECG changes are downsloping and horizontal ST segment depression of 1 mm and more at j point. In ischaemia in angina pectoris it is mostly 2.3 mm horizontal, ST segment depressions noted in more than 2 sets of leads.** It disappears after pain is relieved (Figs 6.2 and 6.3). In many cases ST segment reverses to an isoelectric state within 3 hours (Fig. 6.4).
2. In acute angina ST segment depression 2–3 mm downsloping with t wave inversion V_4, V_5, V_6 (Fig. 6.5).
3. In many cases of IHD with angina (25%) especially in cases of **diabetes mellitus and old age >> 70 years age group**, no ST segment depression is seen. So one has to depend on other signs of disease.
4. A good 12 lead ECG is recorded by a trained ECG technician in the Doctor's office who should read it immediately.

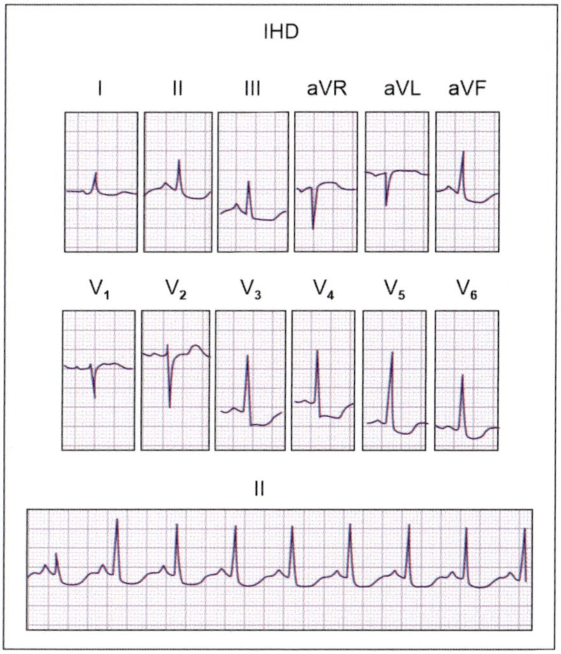

Fig. 6.2: 2–3 mm horizontal, ischaemic ST segment depression in a case of fresh angina pectoris. I, III, AVF, V_3, V_4, V_5, V_6

6

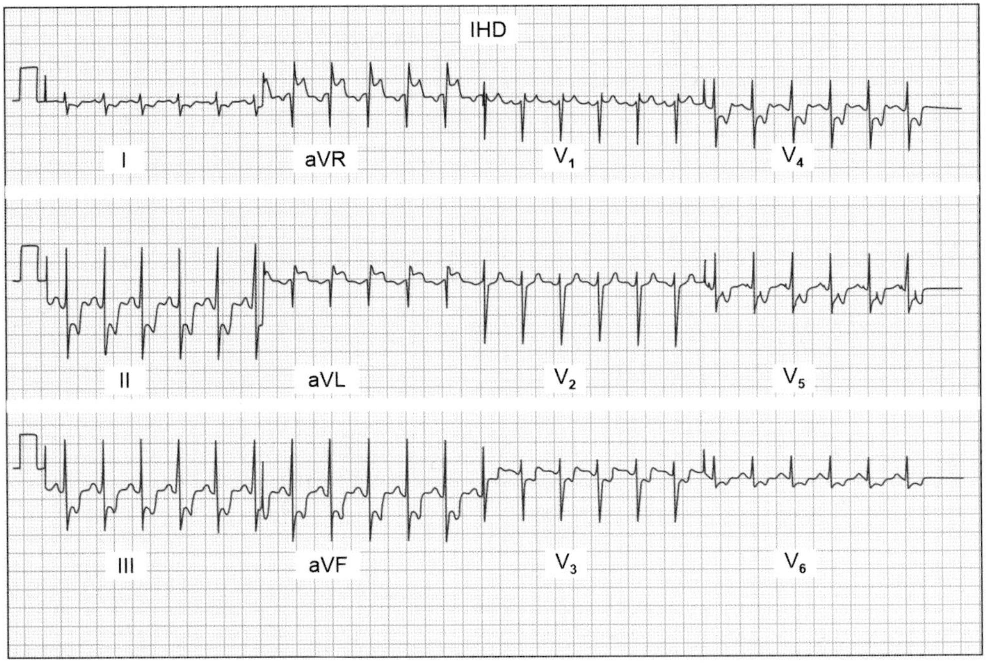

Fig. 6.3: ECG–2.5 mm horizontal ST segment with → sinus tachycardia depression in II, III, aVF, V_3, V_4, V_5

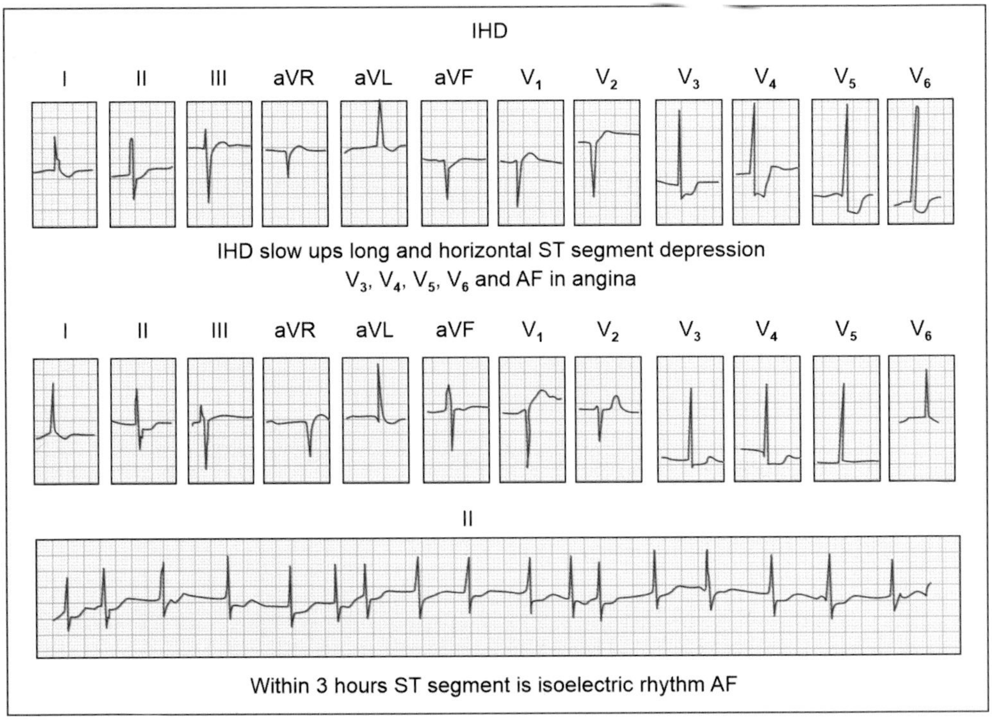

Fig. 6.4: Horizontal ST segment depression in V_3,V_4,V_5,V_6, becomes isolectric within 3 hours rhythm AF persists

6

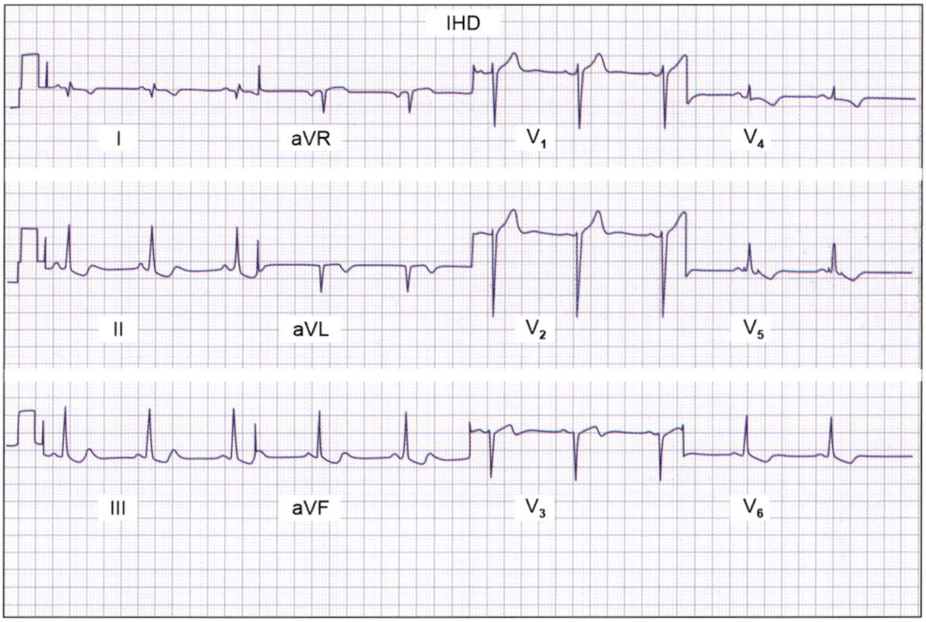

Fig. 6.5: Acute angina—case ST segment depression 2–3 mm (downsloping) II, III, aVF, V_4, V_5, V_6 with T wave inversion V_4, V_5, V_6

5. **T waves changes in angina**
   a. In some cases, we only see symmetrical T wave inversion in certain leads, I, II, III, aVF, V_5, V_6 (Fig. 6.6), or only in pre-cordial leads V_3 to V_6 (Fig. 6.7). The T wave inversion is from 2 to 5 mm and it may disappear after the relief of angina.
   b. ST segment depression and T wave inversion in the same lead during angina pain are also common.

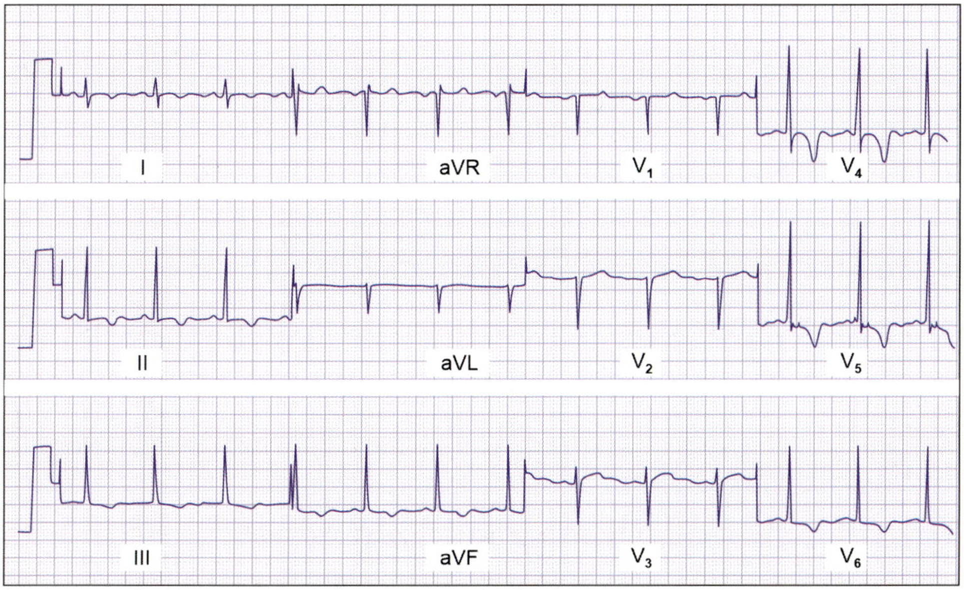

Fig. 6.6: Symmetrical T wave inversion, I, II, III, aVF, V_4, V_5, V_6

6

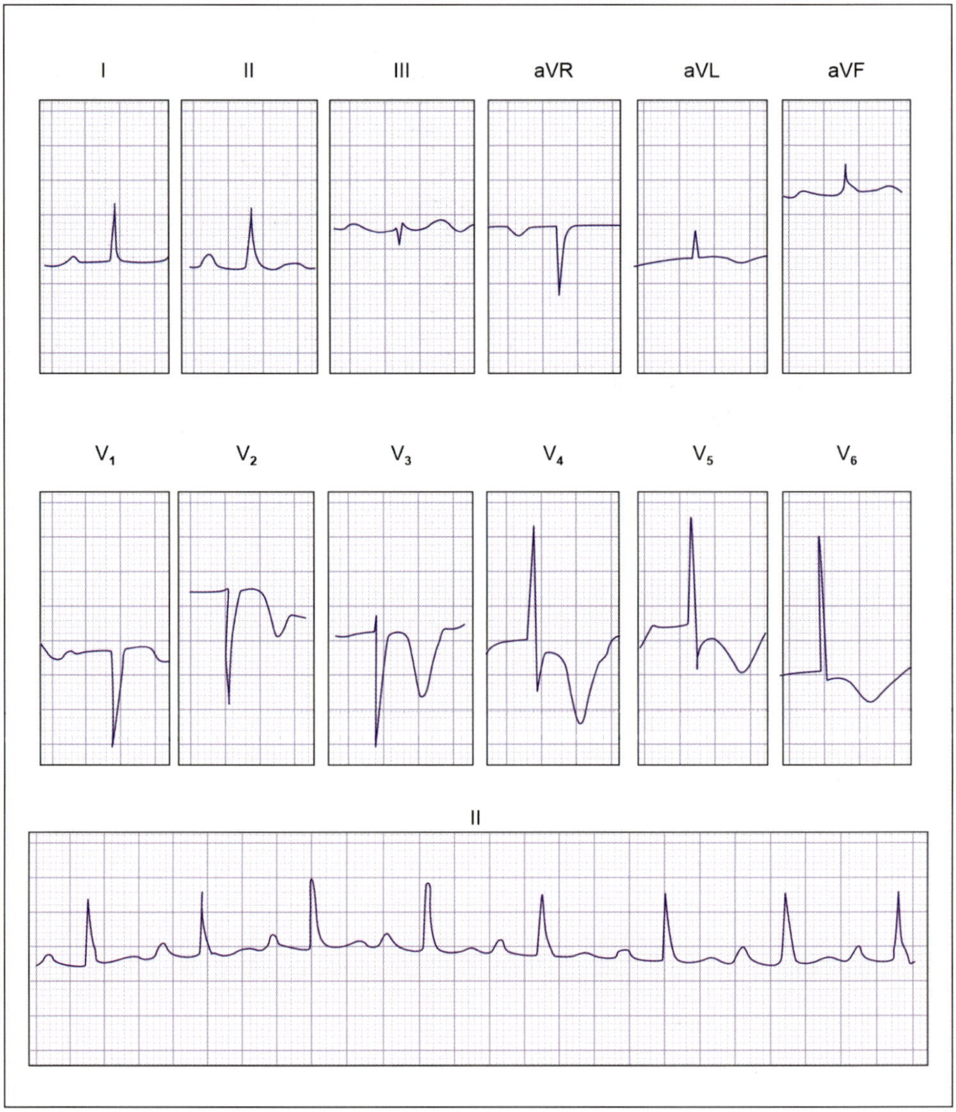

Fig. 6.7: Angina pectoris: Deep symmetrical T wave inversion V_2, V_3, V_4, V_5

6. In old case of MI Q wave seen and with fresh angina, T wave inversion may be the only sign.
7. Rarely during angina many multiple VPC and VT may be recorded with ischaemia disappearing after the pain is relieved. It can be detected by Holter ECG monitor (Fig. 6.8).
8. During angina sometimes Holter ECG recording shows episodes of **ventricular tachycardia transient** (Fig. 6.9a).
9. **Giant T wave inversion in unstable angina** (Fig. 6.9b).

Please *see* ECGs and attached footnotes in Fig. 6.9b.

ST segment depression can be due to many other causes which must be excluded before diagnosing the case as angina pectoris with positive ECG changes.

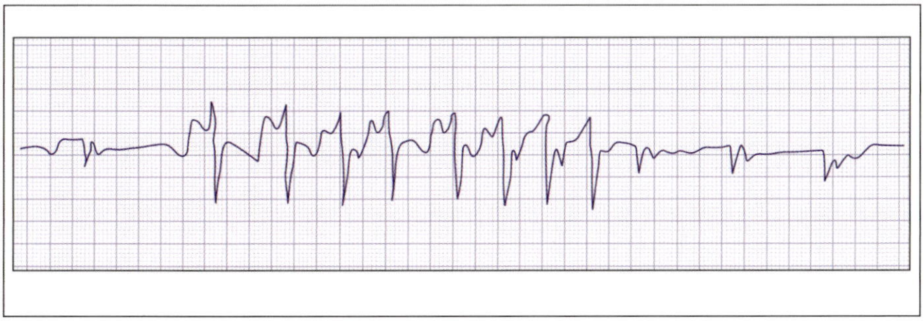

Fig. 6.8: ECG Holter monitor record showing transient myocardial ischaemia

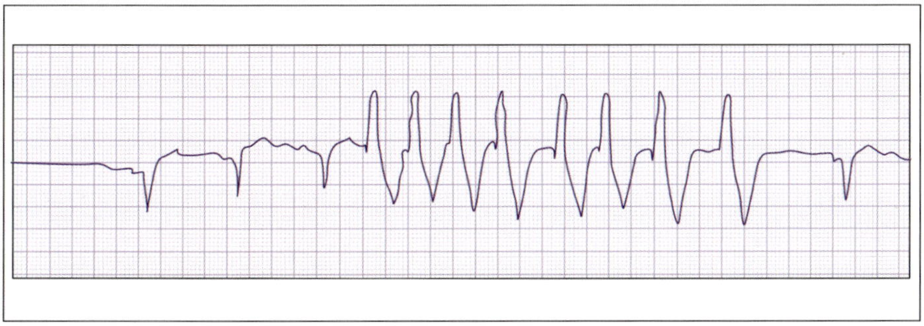

Fig. 6.9a: ECG Holter monitor, transient episode of ventricular tachycardia in angina

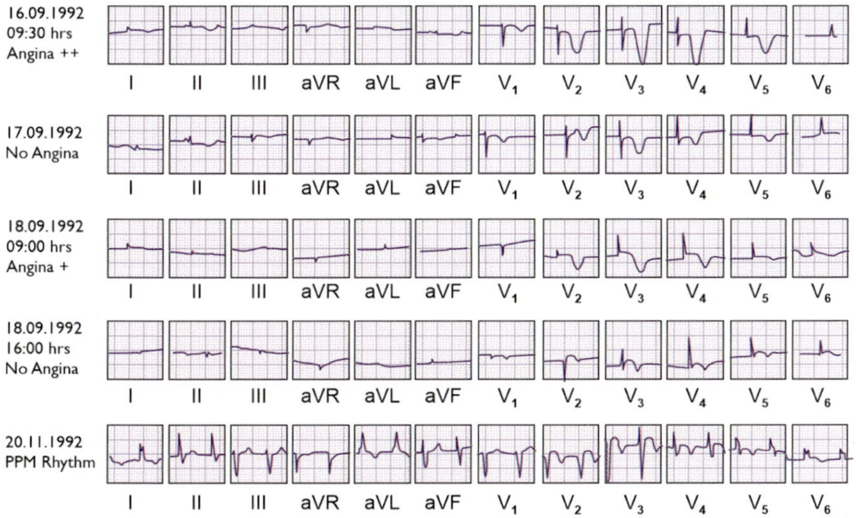

Fig. 6.9b: Unstable angina—giant T wave inversion in precordial leads (V_2, V_3, V_4)

A 45 years old Civilian labourer (low socioeconomic status) developed recurrent unstable angina in two episodes recorded in hospital stay, 16 Sep 1992 to 18 Sep 1992, up to Nov 1992 close follow up. Note: In two episodes of angina ECG showed giant **T wave inversion in V_2, V_3, V_4**, reverting to original state in 24–48 hours after pain relief. No evidence of myocardial necrosis (no trop T ↑). Patient too poor to afford coronary angiography and PTCA even on concession. He developed complete heart block for which hospital provided **free permanent Pacemaker, Nov 1992**.

On telephonic conversation and his yearly visit to hospital at Mangalore till Dec 1998, he had no chest pain. No angina. He was no diabetic and non-hypertensive. He was advised: Tab. aspirin 75 mg OD, tab. metoprolol 25 mg BD and tab NTG 2.6 mg 1 BD (1 tablet twice a day).

Differential Diagnosis of ST Segment1 Depression

Secondary ST segment depression downsloping is also seen in:

a. LBBB: Lead I, aVL, V_4, VS
b. RBBB: Lead V_1, V_2 } Already shown in Chapter 5
c. LVH: I, aVL, V_4, V_5, V_6
d. RVH: V_1, V_2
e. Hyperkalaemia, hypercalcaemia
f. **Acute myocarditis** in all leads
g. Cardiac trauma-direct hit on chest wall-vehicle accidents
h. LV tumour
i. During cardioversion of fatal arrhythmias
j. WPW syndrome
k. Cardiomyopathy.

In a to k. It is not Horizontal ST Segment Depression

In those cases having anginal pain with negative resting ECG we use stress tests in the cardiac laboratory. These tests are:

1. ECG stress test (Fig. 6.10). In this patient is subjected to walk on a **Treadmill** to increase his heart rate mostly up to 120 to 160 per min depending on his height and weight. In this procedure, ECG is simultaneously recorded during exercise. If horizontal ST segment depression of more than 2 mm is noted or patient gets anginal pain then the stress test is stopped immediately (Fig. 6.11). In the olden days before 1965 when modern Stress test was not available we used a double-step wooden table called DMT test. In this test patient used to step up and down at a speed of steps calculated as per his/her age and ECG was recorded immediately and after 3 mts and 6 mts.
2. In one such test, the patient had immediately chest pain in 1 to 2 minutes. ECG recorded showed 4 mm ST segment depression (Fig. 6.12).

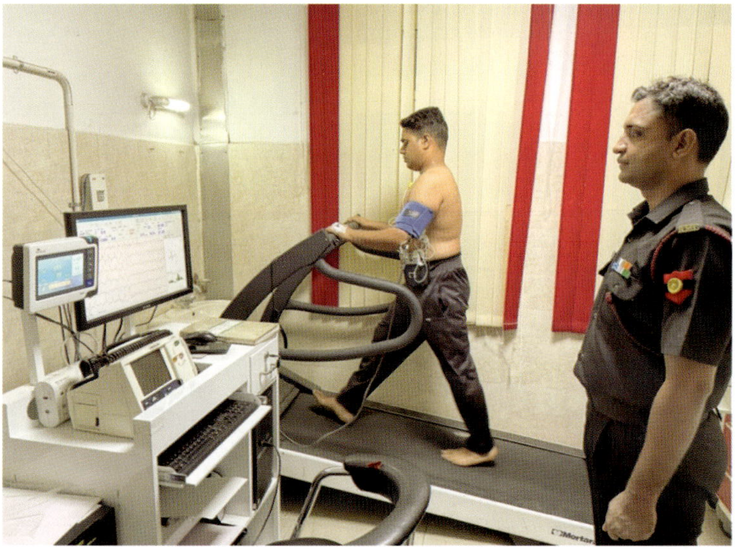

Fig. 6.10: ECG stress test

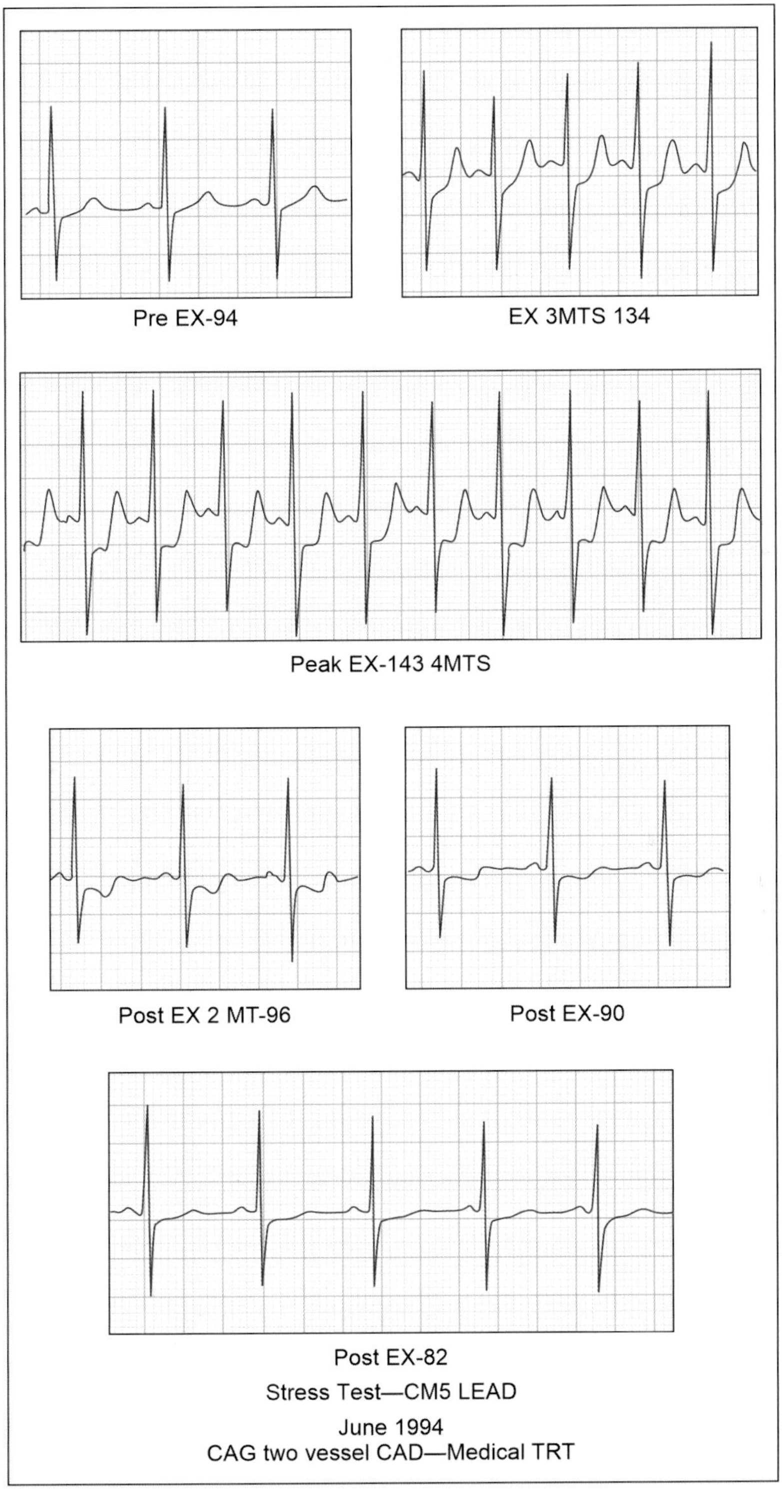

Fig. 6.11: Angina pectoris

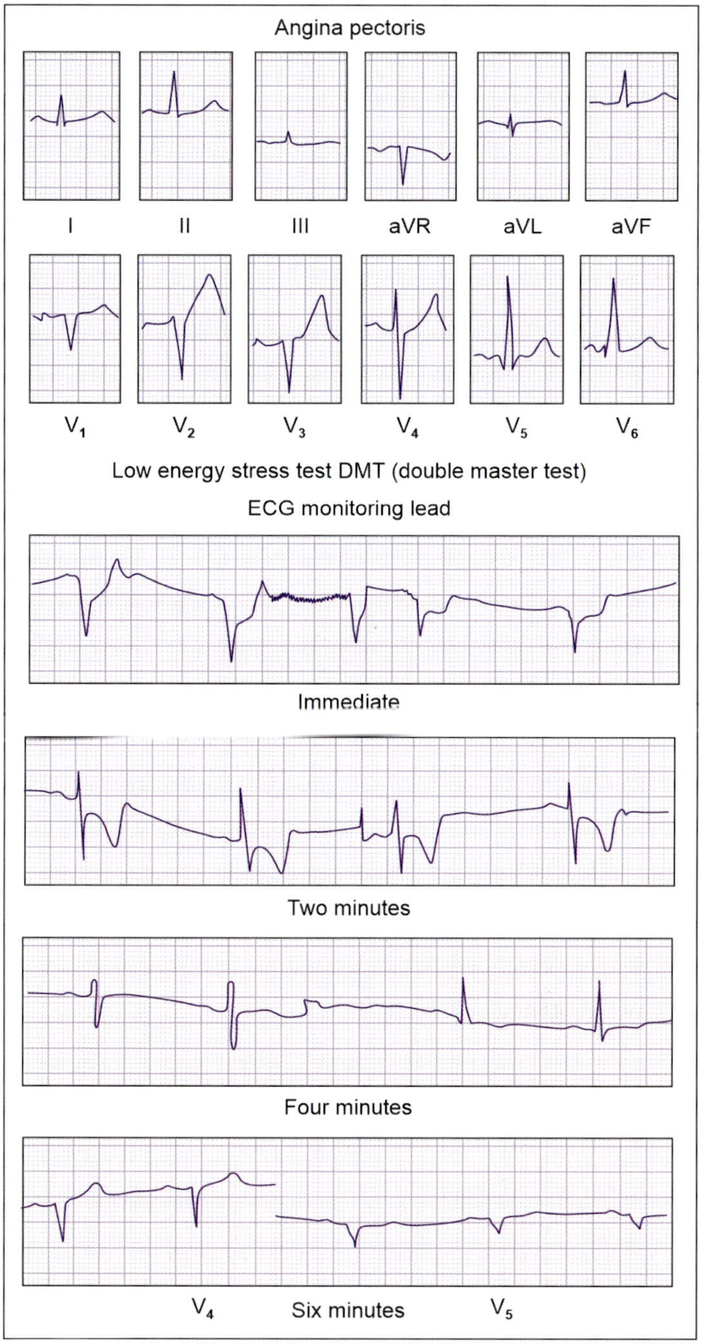

Fig. 6.12: ECG record while doing DMT (Double Master Test)

3. If patient cannot walk due to orthopaedic problem then he is requested to do **static cycling** (cycle ergometry).
4. This patient who cannot cycle then heart rate is increased by injecting dopamine/dobutamine and ECG recorded.

We also have facilities in modern cardiology centres to do the following tests:

1. Stress echocardiography which shows regional wall motion abnormality due to segmental myocardial ischaemia
2. Stress thallium test
3. Stress test used also in rehabilitation post-MI cases (Fig. 6.13)
4. CT contrast angiography
5. And finally contrast coronary angiography which is a gold standard test to diagnose or **exclude coronary atherosclerosis**.

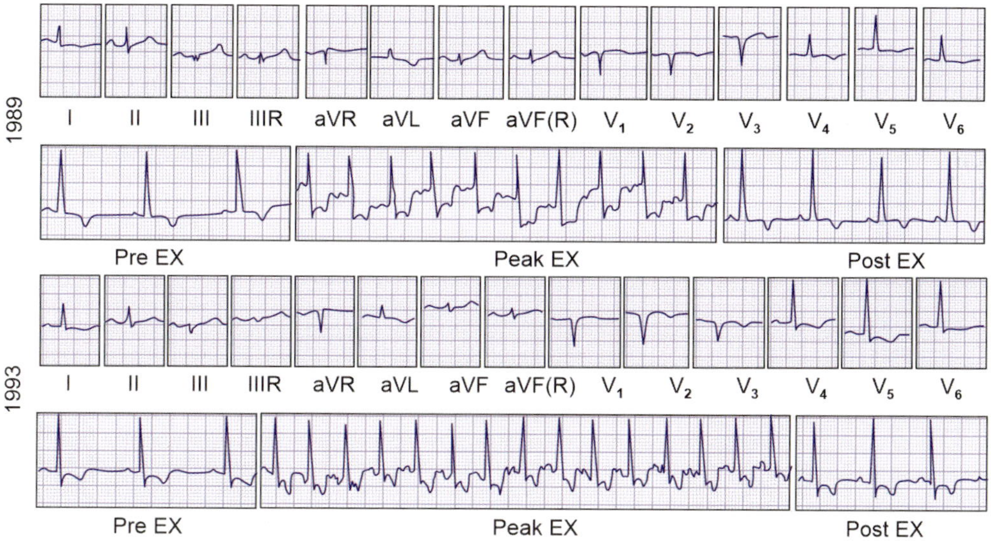

Fig. 6.13: Anteroseptal myocardial infarction four years follow up a symptomatic ECG stress test still positive in rehabilitation after acute MI

Diagnostic Criteria for Vasospastic Angina

1. **Nitrate-responsive angina:** During spontaneous episode, with at least 1 of the following:
   a. Rest angina, especially between night and early morning.
   b. Marked diurnal variation in exercise tolerance, reduced in morning.
   c. Hyperventilation can precipitate an episode.
   d. Calcium channel blockers (not beta blockers) suppress episodes.
2. **Transient ischemic electrocardiographic changes:** During spontaneous episode, including any of the following in at least 2 contiguous leads:
   a. ST segment elevation $\geq$0.1 mV
   b. ST segment depression $\geq$0.1 mV
   c. New negative U waves.
3. **Coronary artery spasm:** Defined as transient total or subtotal coronary artery occlusion (>90% constriction) with angina and ischemic electrocardiographic changes either spontaneously or in response to a provocative stimulus (typically acetylcholine, ergot, or hyperventilation).

6

Practical Aspects of Management

As angina pectoris has many risk factors. These are also evaluated in a patient before finalising his/her treatment. The risk factors are:

Non-modifiable	*Modifiable*
Age	Dyslipidaemia
Male gender	Hypertension
Family history of IHD	Abdominal obesity
Presence of old IHD	Smoking
Physical inactivity	Diabetes
	Diet

For identification of risk factors and checking the patient's overall health status certain laboratory investigations are essential in each case before finalising the line of treatment.

Laboratory Investigations

Blood

1. Complete haemogram
2. CPK, CPKMB, troponin T estimation
3. RFT blood urea, serum creatinine urine RE
4. LFT serum bilirubin, SGOT, SGPT, serum proteins, albumin, globulin and serum amylase.
5. Serum electrolytes—sodium, potassium and magnesium, estimation
6. Serum myoglobin estimation
7. Blood uric acid level
8. Portable–echocardiography for assessment of RWMA, LV wall motion abnormalities, LVEF, any other cardiac abnormality.
9. X-ray heart (portable)
10. ECG daily atleast twice a day
11. Portable Holter ECG monitor if any arrhythmia like VPC, AF, noted on ECG monitor or ST segment changes.
12. Fasting blood sugar
13. Lipid profile
14. Portable echocardiogram at bed side by expert cardiologist twice a day for 3 days to detect mechanical cardiac chamber complications like aneurysm or rupture.

Chronic Coronary Disease

In recent 2023 memorandum on management of ischemic heart disease (chronic coronary disease: CCD). CCD—Concept of shared decision is discussed.

It envolves two parties

a. Clinical care team composed of
   i. Treating cardiologist/physician
   ii. Patient educational expert

   iii. Nutritional expert (dietician)
   iv. Physical activity expert
   v. Experts who treat risk factor of disease, e.g. weight reduction, exercise training, BP control, etc.

b. Patient and his close family members
   i. Level of health literacy of patient
   ii. Level of social economy support
   iii. Level of insurance for medical treatment
   iv. Patient work place environment
   v. Profession of the patient and family responsibilities.

All these factors are discussed and whatever doubts of patient and relatives about his disease are explained in language they understand. Patient impressed with need for his life style change and medical treatment for whole of his life. Patient should have cooperative attitude. All options of treatment for CCD/IHD are available in our country; this point is explained to the patient and his relatives.

General Advice to Patients with Stable Angina

1. Do not smoke
2. Aim for an ideal body weight
3. Take regular exercise (exercise up to, but not beyond, the point of chest discomfort is beneficial and may promote collateral vessels).
4. Avoid severe unaccustomed exertion and vigorous exercise after a heavy meal or in very cold weather.
5. Take rest for half an hour after each meal.

Reduction of weight by following exercise program and in the diet scheme the following advice is given. These should be strictly followed by the patient.

a. The fat content of the food the saturated fat like ghee, coconut oil, etc. should contribute only 6% of the calories. Patient can take one day a week saturated fat preparation like prantha, dosas (cooked in coconut oil. Main contribution of the fat should be from polysaturated fat (51% of daily calories pr monosaturated fat 50% of the daily calories from the fat component. So patient should take olive oil Sunola, Saffola, Rice bran oil.
b. Carbohydrates and proteins: Green vegetables and fresh fruits, whole multi grain Atta (In 5 kg wheat atta ½ kg each of, Saffola, black gram, bajra and Jaoin should be mixed. This atta should be used for daily preparation of chapattis. Brown bread instead of white bread should be used.
c. Protein contents should be from lean non fatty meat, e.g. chicken, birds. No fried preparations should be taken. Avoid sugar sweetened beverages. No baked precooked food.
d. Alcoholic preparation should be avoided. The cardiac cases with documented cardiac muscle damage and/or with LVEF <40% alcohol intake is totally prohibited.
e. Total sodium content of daily food should be <2300 mg, total potassium should be 3500 mg per day. Avoid extra salt at the dining table.

f. The use of readymade **Nutrition Supplement** is highlighted on TV, Mobile, and Internet and Print media daily for preventing heart attack (Unchecked and Uncontrolled). This has been disproved by the 2023 guidelines with the statement, **"In patients with CCD, the use of nonprescription or dietary supplements, including Omega-3 fatty acid, vitamins C, D, E, BETA-Carotene, and Calcium is not beneficial to reduce the risk of acute CVD events.**

g. To keep the ideal level of LDL Cholesterol 70 mg %, patients are advised statin therapy for whole life. Statins with >50% lowering capacity of LDL like **Atorvostatin** 20–40 mg OD/**Rousvastatin** 20–40 mg should be used. Other statin preparation like Simvastatin, Prvavastatin, Lovastatin, Fluvastatin, Pitvavastatin should be avoided.

Blood pressure control: Blood pressure is an important risk factor of **IHD**. It should be kept between 100/70 to 130/80 mm hg. Beside the drugs treatment Nonpharmacologic Strategies for blood pressure management are advised which are:

1. Regular walking Aerobic exercise 20–30 minutes per daily to achieve the heart rate increase to 100–110 per minutes.
2. Avoided isometric exercises like hand grip, weight lifting, etc. to be avoided, as they increased LVEDP (LV end diastolic pressure) more than 20 mmHg, which is very harmful in cases of heart disease.
3. Should reduce weight and keep ideal weight for his age and sex by diet control and exercise.
4. He should take healthy diet prefebary DASH dietary pattern–consume a diet rich in fruits, vegetables, whole grains, and low fat dairy products, with reduced content of saturated and total fat.
5. Never use trans fat (Repeatedly heating the same oil for frying samosha and meat preparation.

Recommendations for sexual health and activity. In patients with CCD cardiac rehabilitation and regular exercise can be useful to reduce the risk of cardiovascular complications with sexual activity. In the male patients who use phosphodiesterase type 5 inhibitors for improving penis errection should not be allowed to take nitrate medication because of risk for severe hypotension DASH (dietary approaches to stop hypertension).

Drugs Treatment

- Following groups of drugs are used in the management of angina pectoris:
  - Nitrates
  - β-adrenergic receptor antagonists (β-blockers)
  - Calcium antagonists
  - Platelet inhibitors
  - Miscellaneous (ranolazine, trimetazidine, and ivabradine).
  - Anti-diabetic drug SGLT2 inhibitors and GLP-1 receptor agonists as per recommendation of 2023 guidelines of AHA/ACC for use in IHD cases with diabetes mellitus even, in some non diabetic patients they are proved usefull.

Nitrates

6

- **Glyceryl trinitrate (GTN)** acts by venous and arteriolar dilatation, which lowers blood pressure, reduces venous return to heart, and dilates coronary vessels. By producing vasodilation, end-diastolic subendocardial perfusion increases.

- **Fresh glyceryl trinitrate (5 mg) sublingually relieves pain in 2–3 minutes** and produces mild headache. Patient is instructed to spit out or swallow the tablet once pain is relieved.
- The best use of GTN is prophylactically before exercise known to produce pain.
- Not more than three tablets per hour should be used. Use of GTN should be encouraged because physical activity promotes the formation of collateral vessels.
- **Tablet TNG (Trinitroglycerin) extended release 2.6 mg** twice a day is also a very useful treatment for angina.
- **Isosorbide dinitrate** has prolonged action (10–20 mg two to three times a day) and is given orally. It can also be given sublingually. Headache is a common side effect. Tolerance develops and the dose needs to be increased. It is important to have a 10 to 12 hours nitrate-free period to avoid tolerance. Hence, doses are given in the **morning and afternoon**.
- Isosorbide mononitrate needs to be given once or twice a day.
- **Long-acting nitrates** are often used if symptoms are not controlled with β-blockers and/or calcium channel blockers. Although there is no evidence that nitrates improve patient prognosis, long-acting nitrates reduce the frequency and severity of angina attacks in patients with stable angina.
- **Contraindications to nitrate treatment**
  1. HOCM
  2. Severe aortic stenosis
  3. Constrictive pericarditis
  4. Mitral stenosis
  5. Close angle glaucoma.

Beta-Blockers

- They reduce myocardial oxygen demand by reducing heart rate for a given level of exercise, reducing heart rate response. In addition, because of their negative chronotropic effect, β-blockers prolong diastole, prolonging coronary artery blood flow, and myocardial perfusion.
- Cardioselective β-blockers. These include metoprolol (50–200 mg/day) and atenolol (50–200 mg/day).
- **Carvedilol** (3.125–25 mg twice a day) has additional unique effects that include, its antiarrhythmic effects, antioxidant and antiproliferative properties that inhibit apoptosis.
- **Carvedilol is the best β-blocker drug to be prescribed now**, Metoprolol/Atenolol had their days in last 2 decades.
- β-blockers should not be withdrawn abruptly as there is a risk of dangerous arrhythmias and myocardial infarction. This occurs due to up-regulation of β-adrenergic receptors when patients are treated with β-blockers.
- **Absolute contraindications** to β-blockers are severe bradycardia, conduction system disease (sinus node dysfunction and/or high-grade AV block), bronchial asthma, peripheral vascular disease, and depression.
- Prinzmetal's angina may worsen with β-blockers due to an unopposed β-adrenergic effect.

Calcium Channel Blockers

- Mode of action. **They inhibit the flow of slow in-ward current caused by the entry of extracellular calcium through cell membrane of excited cells, particularly in SA node, AV node, and ventricular muscle-based ectopic, cardiac atrial cells and arterioles**. Dilatation of peripheral arteries reduces blood pressure (afterload), thereby reducing myocardial workload, and reducing oxygen requirement.
- Amlodipine and felodipine, produce coronary and peripheral arterial dilatation. Verapamil and diltiazem in addition reduce conductivity.
- Verapamil is given at a dose of 40–80 mg TDS, main side effect is constipation. **This drug is not very much used these days**. When used with β-blockers it can cause CCF due to marked negative ionotropic effect on the cardiac muscles.
- Since β-blockers have been shown to reduce mortality after myocardial infarction, it is reasonable to start a β-blockers and then add a calcium channel blocker if required. It is better to avoid this combination.
- Calcium blockers are indicated in patients with inadequate response to β-blockers, COPD cases and cases of peripheral vascular disease. In addition to cases of sick sinus syndrome and AV block.

Antiplatelet Agents

In this group of drugs for angina, aspirin and clopidogrel are mainly used. These drugs are more commonly used in cases of IHD after coronary intervention, e.g. PTCA with stent application. Those cases of angina that do not respond to anti-anginal drugs, require coronary intervention procedures to be discussed in next pages.

Miscellaneous Drugs

a. **Angiotensin-converting enzyme inhibitors**, like ramipril are used in angina when there is associated CCF or LHF. Before their use please check blood urea and serum creatinine. (If blood urea more than 50 mg % and or serum creatinine more than 2 mg%) these drug should not be used.
    - In patients with CCD who also have hypertension, diabetes, with LVEF is 40% or less and CKD cases, the use of ACE indhibitors, or ARBs if ACE inhibitor-intolerant, is recommended to reduce cardiovascular events. In those cases where LVEF >40% the use of ACE inhibitors or ARBs may be considered to reduce cardiovascular events.

b. **Ranolazine** is a late sodium ion channel inhibitor, by preventing intracellular sodium overload. There is more diastolic muscle relaxation and oxygen requirement is reduced. It does not affect heart rate and blood pressure. It can be safely used in cases of bradycardia and hypotension, dose 500 to 1000 mg bd. Initially for a few weeks and then once a day.

c. **Ivabradine:** Selectively inhibits in-ward sodium-potassium current, an important pacemaking current in a SA node. It lowers the heart rate and it is useful in patients of angina with tachycardia it can be combined with other drugs dose 5 mg BD.

d. **Trimetazidine:** It is a cardiac muscle cell metabolic modulator, that improves its oxygen-utilizing capacity and glucose metabolism. It increases coronary flow reserve, lowers the frequency of angina episodes, improves exercise performance and spares the use of nitrates without any changes in the heart. It can be used with other drugs.

e. **Anti diabetic drugs use in IHD**

For use of SGLT2 inhibitors and GLP-1 receptor agonists (anti diabetic drugs).

Latest recommendation: In patients with CCD and type 2 diabetes, addition of a GLP-1 receptor agonist is projected to be of high value compared with the previous accepted standard of care. In patients with CCD and heart failure with LVEF ≤40%, use of an SGLT2 inhibitor is recommended to reduce the risk of cardiovascular death and heart failure hospitalization and to improve QOL, irrespective of diabetes status. In patients with CCD and heart failure with LVEF >40%, use of an SGLT2 inhibitor can be beneficial in decreasing heart failure hospitalizations and to improve QOL, irrespective of diabetes status.

Summary of Drug Therapy for Angina in CCD (Chronic Coronary Artery Disease)

- **Baseline therapy:** Consider aspirin, statin, and ACEI therapy in all patients. Sublingual nitroglycerin as needed.
  Smoking cessation and lifestyle changes.
- **Antianginal Rx**
- **First line: Beta blocker** (e.g. carvedilol 6.25 mg BID uptitrated)
- **Second line: CCB** substituted (non DHP [e.g. Diltiazem 75 mg BID titrated]) where beta blockers are not tolerated or ineffective.
- **Third line: Add-in therapy**
- **CCB-DHP** (e.g. Amlodipine) only for those on beta blockers
- **Nicorandil** (5 mg BID, uptitrated)
- **Ranolazine** (500 mg BID, uptitrated)
- **In diabetes mellitus cases add SGL2 inhibitors and GLP-1 receptor agonists.**

Interventional Therapy—Absolute Indications

This is indicated when the patient does not respond to anti-anginal drug therapy, as discussed in previous paragraphs, or it is absolutely indicated in:

1. Left main stem artery block (LMS disease)
2. Strongly positive stress test
3. Proximal LAD block
4. Patients of younger age groups between 30 and 50 years
5. Patient is not cooperative in his drugs intake regularly.

Interventional therapy is discussed in the subsequent paragraphs, under myocardial infarction.

Acute Myocardial Infarction

This is an acute medical emergency requiring urgent treatment.

Clinical presentation has been discussed earlier in Chapters 1 and 2 of this document. The ECG findings are as follows.

ST Segment Elevation

1. **Classical ST segment elevation** with convexity upwards with tall T wave especially in V_2, V_3 and V_4 leads, is seen in the earliest phases of acute myocardial infarction (Fig. 6.14). This finding disappears in a few hours (4–12 hours), ST segment becomes isoelectric and T wave inversion occurs up to 2–5 mm with in next few days. In two conjugate leads V_2,V_3 or I, II.

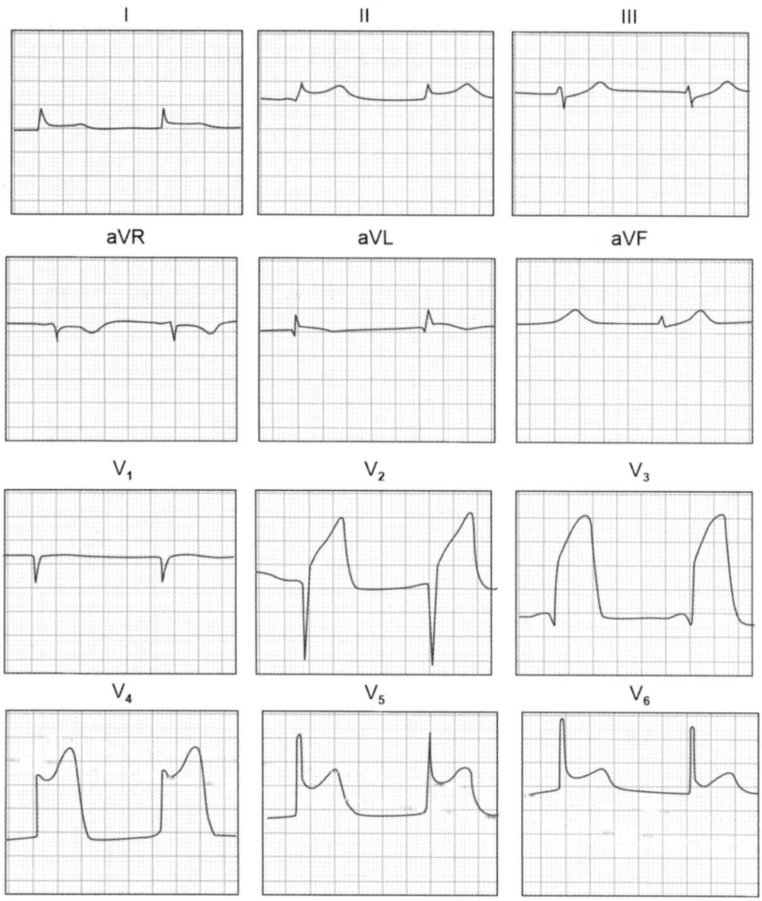

Fig. 6.14: Fresh anterior wall MI hyperacute ST elevation up to 10 mm with tall T wave

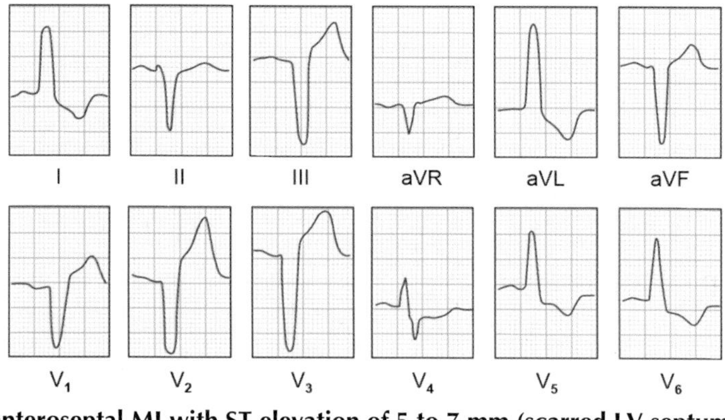

Fig. 6.15: Old anteroseptal MI with ST elevation of 5 to 7 mm (scarred LV septum) (LV aneurysm)

2. **ST segment elevation persisting without MI** is seen in prinzmetal angina due to coronary artery spasm, disappears after pain relief.
3. **ST segment elevation without pain and 2 m↑** convexity upward especially in V_2–V_5 lead is suggestive of scarred myocardium due to old MI (Fig. 6.15).

6

4. **A benign cause of ST segment elevation due to j point elevation** with concavity upwards is seen in Younger people up to 30 years. It is due to early repolarisation and in repeated ECG remains same (Fig. 6.16).

J point elevation causing ST segment—elevation with concavity upwards in the leads V2, V3, V4 is normal finding up to the age of 25 years female in two ECG taken in the gap of one hour same finding persist, this is a normal variation this is due to early repolarisation

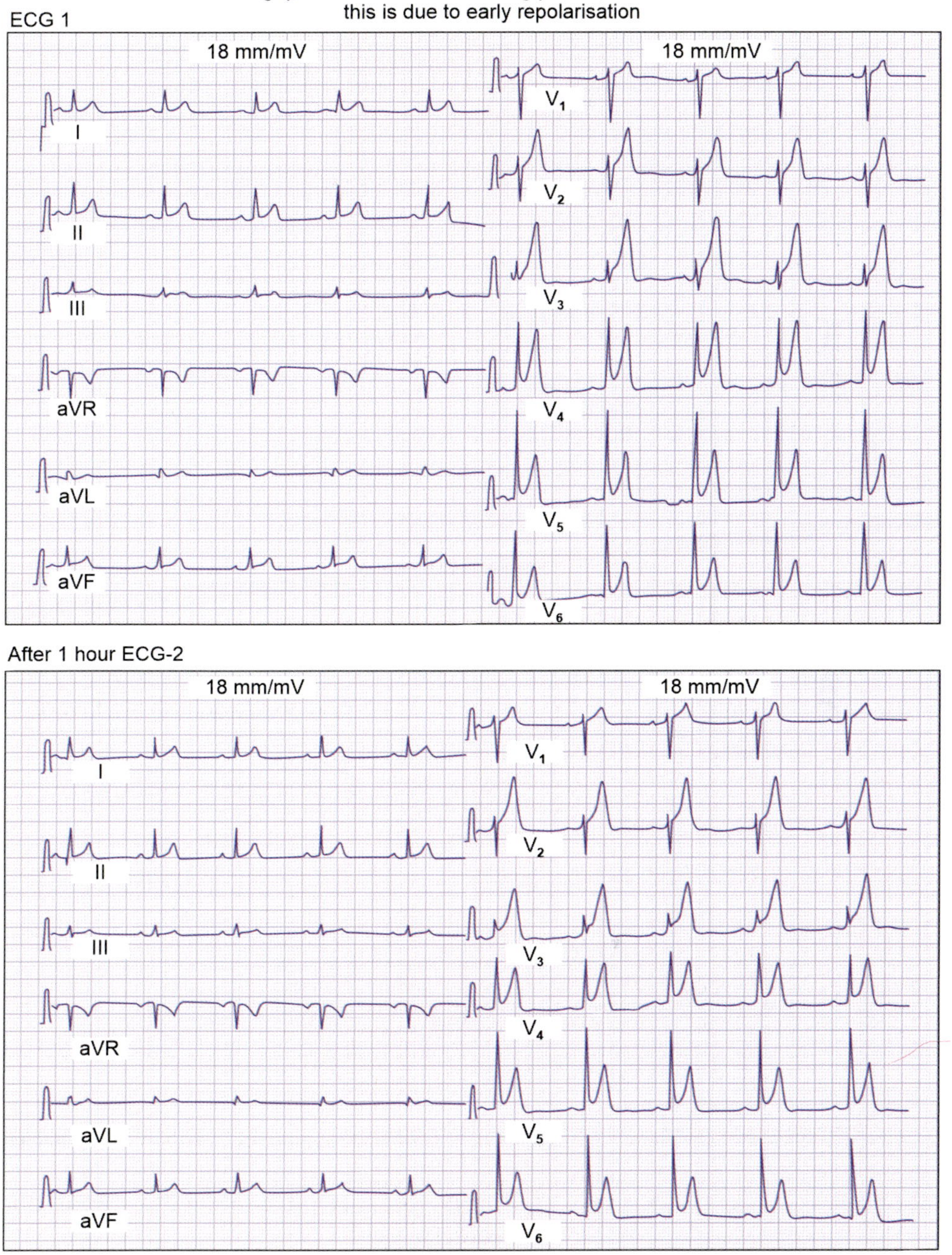

Fig. 6.16

Sequence of ECG Changes in Acute Myocardial Infarction

a. First and foremost is ST ↑↑ 2–8 cm with convexity upward (Fig. 6.14) and hyperacute T wave. It disappears within a few hours and becomes isoelectric in 1–2 days. Earlier if thrombolysis done with STK or tenecteplase (Fig. 6.17).

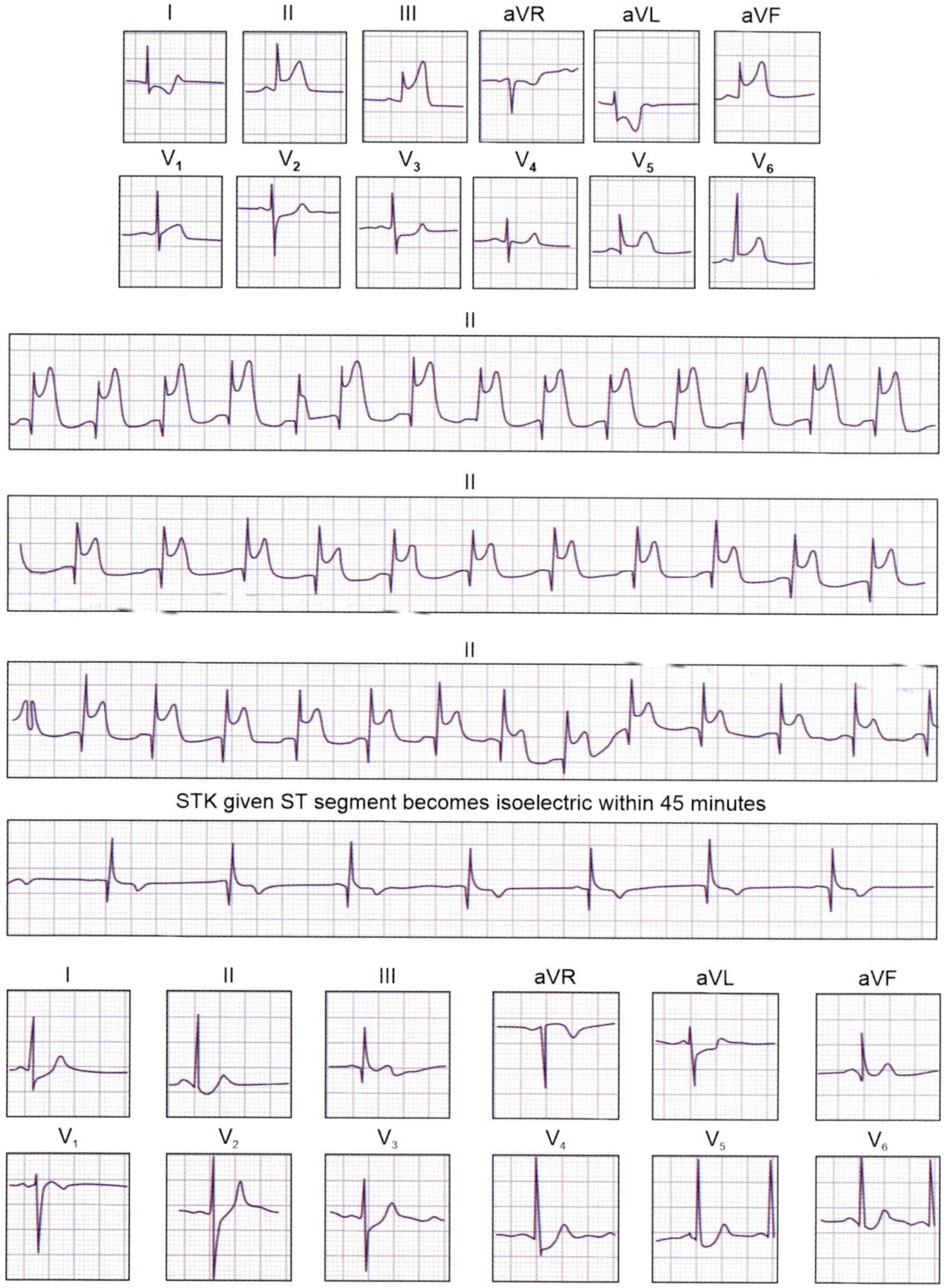

AC inferior wall MI successfully thrombolysed
Fresh inferior wall MI

Fig. 6.17

b. As ST segment becomes, isoelectric, Q wave appears preceding RS wave. Pathological Q wave is more than 0.04 to 0.08 mm in width and has a depth of more than 25% of the next R wave (Fig. 6.18). Even Q waves may merge with S waves giving QS format.

c. **Reciprocal ST segment depression** on the opposite side of LV area, e.g. in inferior wall MI. ST ↑ of II, III, AVF is associated with ST segment depression of V_1, V_4 disappearing in 24 hours (Fig. 6.19). Sometimes the whole process takes **10–11 days** (Fig. 6.20).

d. **Differential diagnosis of pathological Q wave:**
   1. WPW (Fig. 6.21)
   2. Myocarditis

25% of Q waves in inferior wall MI disappear but Q waves of anterior wall MI in precordial leads persist lifelong.

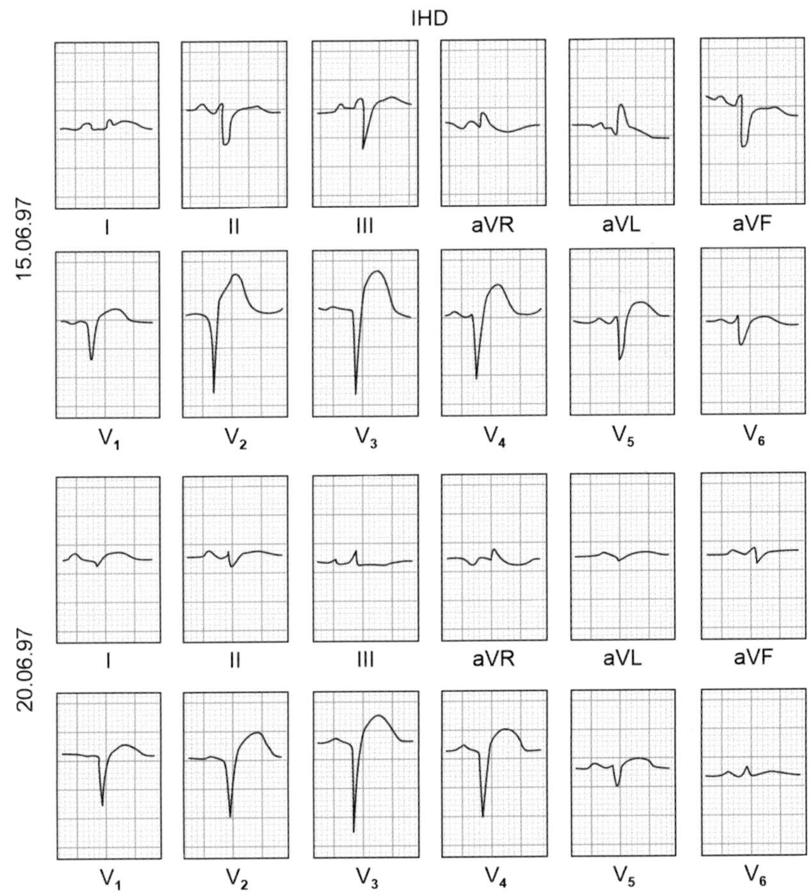

Extensive anterior wall MI-Q in—V_1, V_2, V_3, V_4, V_5

Fig. 6.18

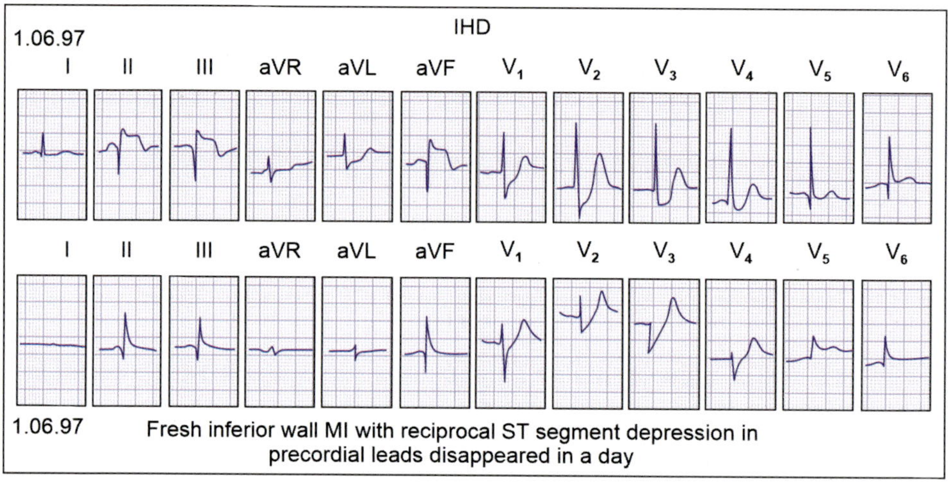

Fig. 6.19: Fresh inferior wall with reciprocal ST segment depression in precordial leads disappeared in a day

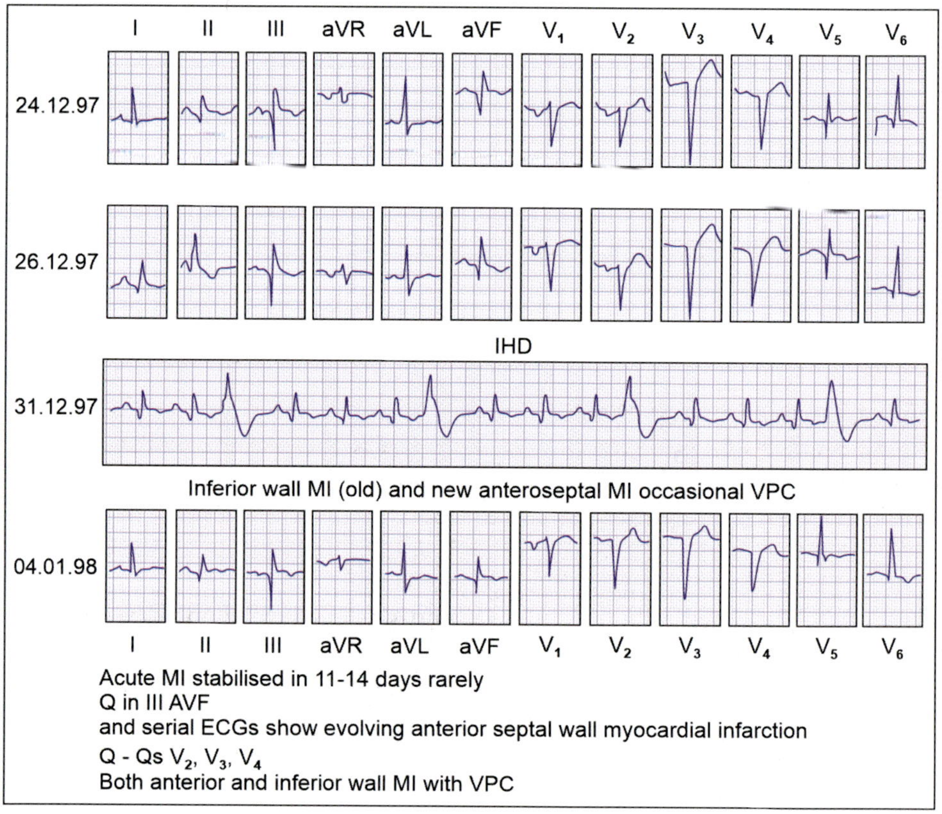

Fig. 6.20: Fresh old inferior wall as MI and fresh anteroseptal MI

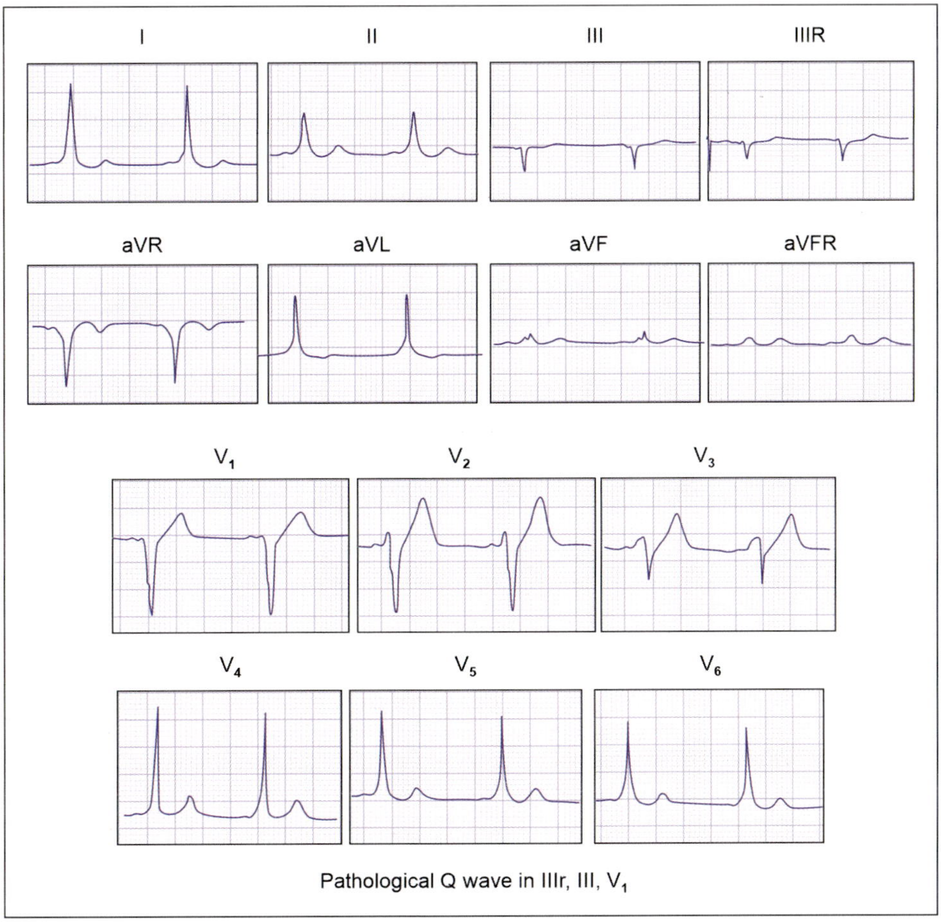

Fig. 6.21: WPW syndrome

Associated T waves Changes in MI

1. **Isolated T wave inversions up to 2 mm** symmetrical in shape up to 2 mm in **lead I, II, III, AVF, AVL, V_3–V_6** are seen in acute MI and it should **persist after the pain is relieved** (Fig. 6.22). If there is associated Troponin T Elevation then it is very significant, indicating myocardial necrosis.
2. In old case of MI Q wave was seen and with fresh chest pain, T wave inversion may be the only sign and signifying myocardial necrosis.
3. Rarely during angina many multiple VPC and VT be recorded on Holter examination, disappearing after pain (Fig. 6.9).
4. Sometimes Holter monitor of ECG is required in cases of angina, especially with microvascular disease it shows silent myocardial ischaemia (Fig. 6.8).
5. T wave inversion **of 2–3 mm or more and symmetrical seen in MI associated with elevated troponin level**.
6. Tall T wave >5 mm or 10 mm is noted in HOCM (Fig. 6.23).

In hyperacute MI-earliest change in precordial leads and more than 7 mm in limb leads. In case of inferolateral MI (Fig. 6.14).

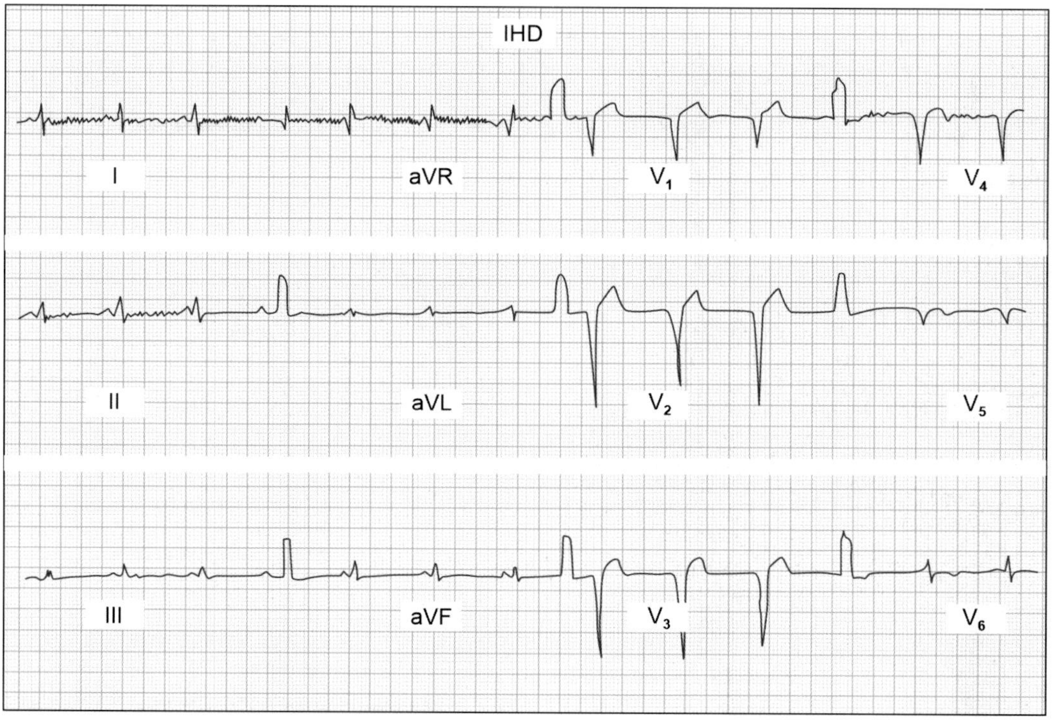

Fig. 6.25: Anterior wall MI (QS in V_1–V_5 in 29 years Youngman) CAG-2VCAD-Being asymptomatic—medical TRT S. triglyceride 550 mg S. cholestrol 240 mg

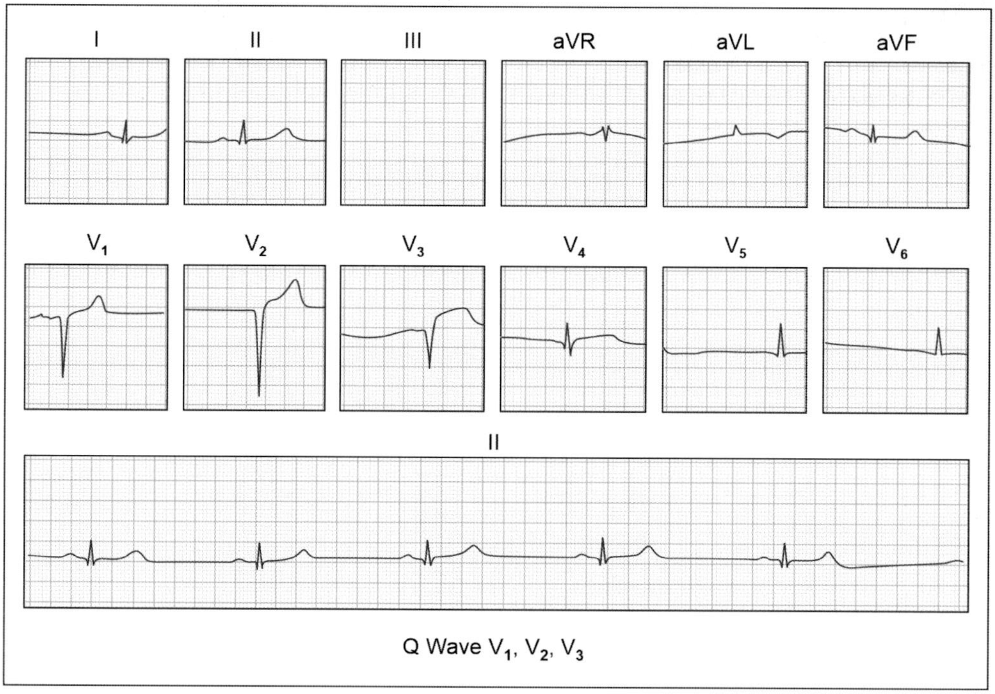

Fig. 6.26a: Antroseptal myocardial infarction

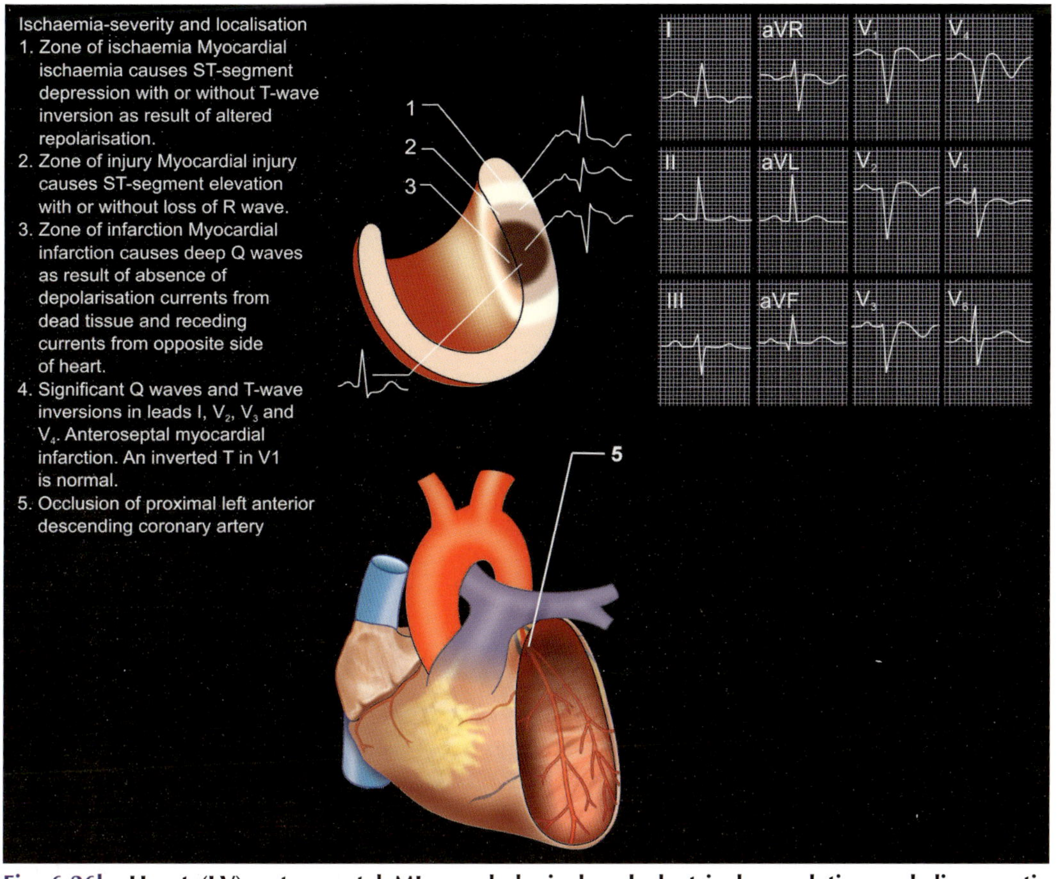

Fig. 6.26b: Heart (LV) anteroseptal MI morphological and electrical correlation and diagramatic representation of ECG changes in Ischemia, injury and MI and Q wave in V_2,V_3,V_4

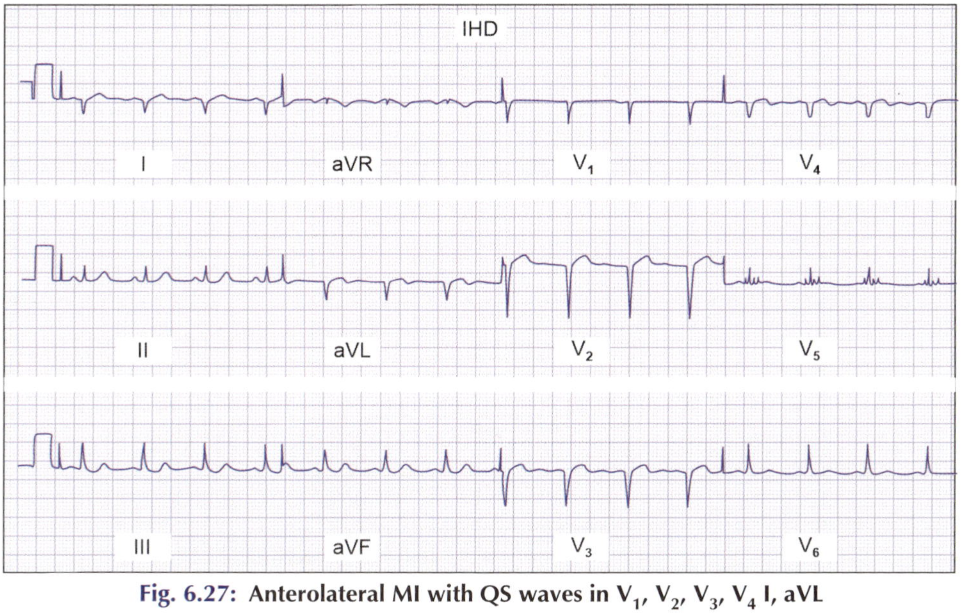

Fig. 6.27: Anterolateral MI with QS waves in V_1, V_2, V_3, V_4 I, aVL

6

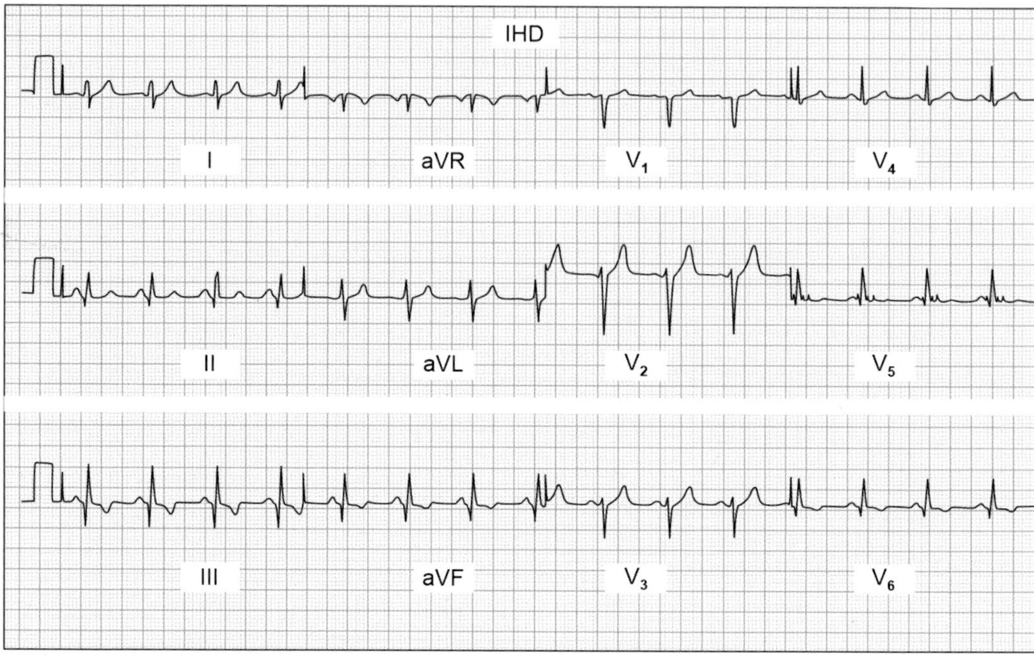

Fig. 6.28: Q in II, III, aVF, old inferior, wall MI

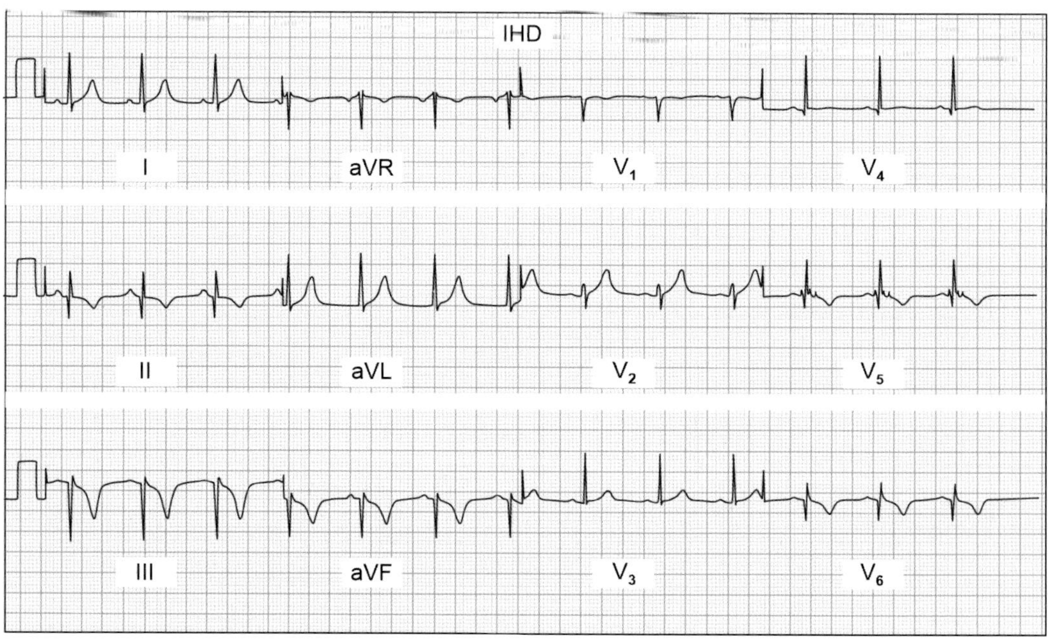

Fig. 6.29: Inferolateral MI Q with deep T wave ↓in III, aVF, V_5, V_6

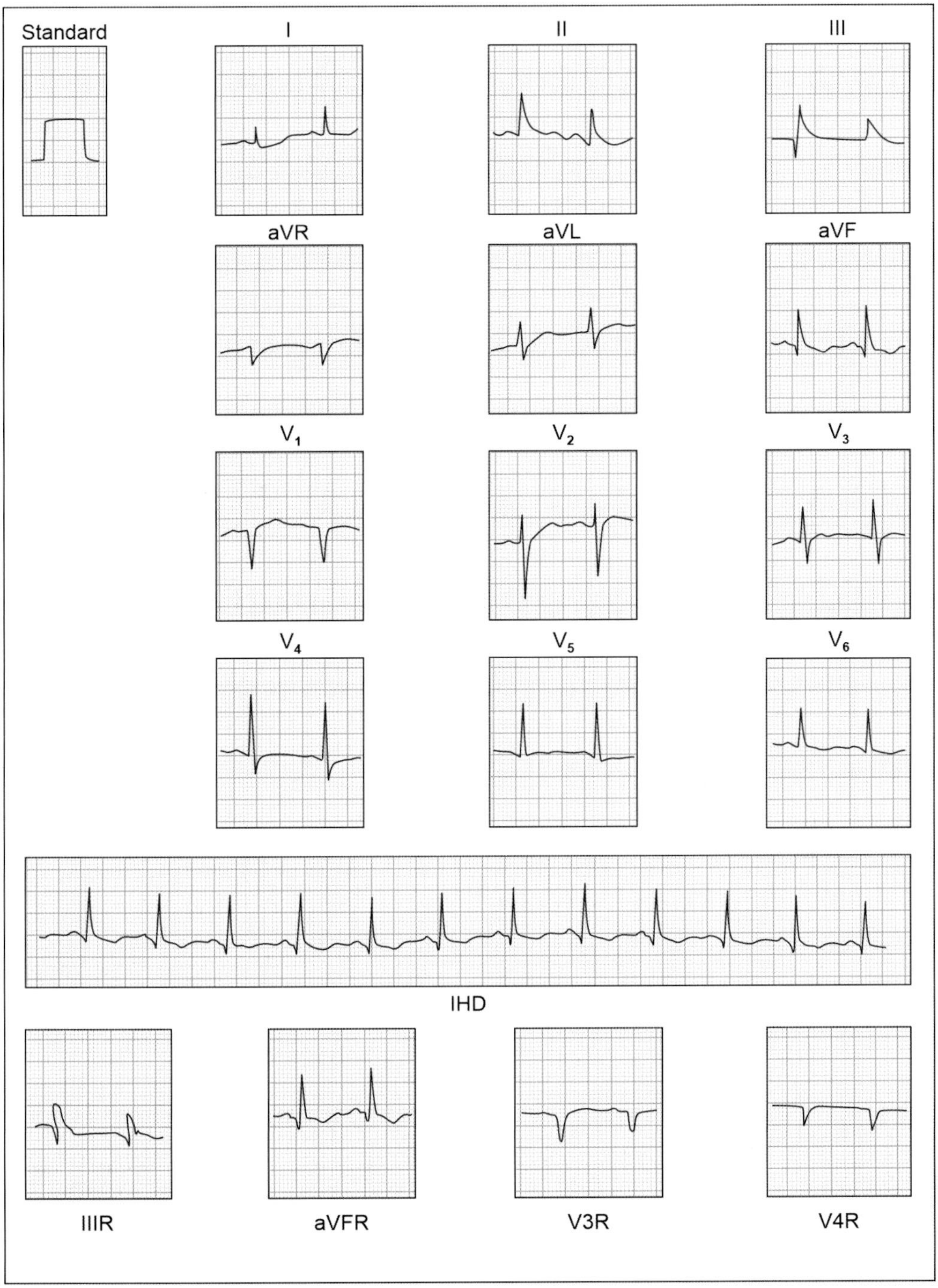

Fig. 6.30: Right ventricle myocardial infarction (Q wave in V_1, V_3R, V_4R, III and IIIR)

Tall R wave in V_1, V_2, V_3, V_4 with ST segment depression in V_2, V_3, V_4, T wave V_4, flat T wave V_5, V_6

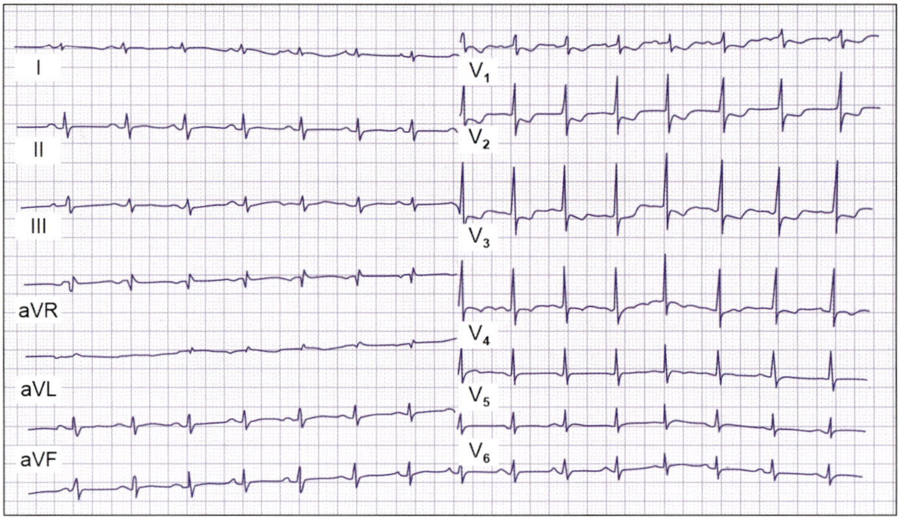

Fig. 6.31a: Posterior myocardial infarction

Acute MI Presenting with VT (Fig. 6.31b)

This patient presented with severe palpitation and retrosternal chest pain and sweating with mild hypotension on 5th May 1974. ECG showed ventricular tachycardia. After treatment with Lignocaine and DC conversion VT was treated but next ECG within ½ hours of hospital admission showed fresh extensive anterior wall myocardial infarction which was treated with the available medicine in 1974 successfully.

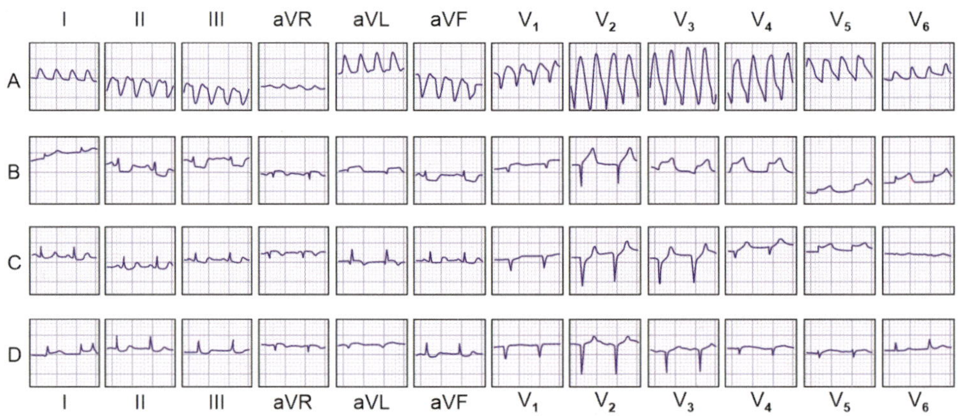

(A) Lead →V_5 show ventricular tachycardia

(B) After 32 minutes ECG pattren of fresh extensive anterior wall MI in lead I a, VL, V_1, V_5

(C) After 28 minutes ST segment becomes almost isoelectric especially in aVL V_2, V_3, V_4 and V_6

(D) After 10 hours ST segment isoelectric in leads aVL V_1, V_2, V_3, V_4, V_5 with pattern of extensive myocardial infarction

Fig. 6.31b: Acute MI presenting as ventricular tachycardia

Practical Emergency Treatment of Acute Myocardial Infarction

Coronary Intervention

Coronary angioplasty (CAG) facilities are now available in all district level hospitals in India and even at block level hospitals in Karnataka, Kerala and parts of Maharashtra and Punjab. **Modern treatment of MI is revascularisation of infarcted area** at the earliest either by IVSTK or IV Tenecteplase and preferably by primary **PTCA (percutaneous transluminal coronary angioplasty)** in Level III hospital if a patient reaches the hospital within a stipulated time of 12 hours after the onset of chest pain. Primary angioplasty is done with stent application (PTCA). For this treatment, the cardiologist should be able to identify affected LV muscle area and the probably occluded coronary artery branch on the critical analysis of surface ECG alone (Appendix 6.1). He should be well-trained in all interventional procedure. After the successful procedure, these patient is shifted to cardiac ICU, where he/she is closely observed by trained nursing and medical staff. After 24–48 hours he/she is shifted to the cardiac ward.

Conventional Treatment of Acute Myocardial Infarction

Thrombolytic treatment, if patient cannot afford level III hospital treatment or cannot reach there in time, then within 12–18 hours IV streptokinase or IV tenecteplase is given. If given within one hour complete thrombolysis of the clot in the coronary artery occurs and ST segment elevation comes down within half an hour to 45 minutes (Fig. 6.17).

Uncomplicated cases of acute MI are kept in cardiac ICU for 1–2 days and then in cardiac ward for 1–2 days more and then discharged home. **Complicated cases with arrhythmias and LVF/stroke** are kept in cardiac ICU for a long time, till they are stable haemodynamically and are self ambulant.

- For relief of pain injection **morphine** 5 mg to 10 mg given IV, can be repeated after 4 hours. If morhine is not available then injection Tramadol 100 mg/2 ml, 6–8 hourly is given. It can be followed by oral capsule Tramadol 50 mg twice a day till the pain is relieved. Patient is put on oxygen for 24–48 hours.
- ECG is continuously monitored in cardiac ICU for cardiac arrhythmias, and with oximetry, BP checkup for 2 days in uncomplicated MI.
- Patient is given aspirin 300 mg, clopidogrel 10 mg immediately, and repeated daily.
- He is also given beta-blocker (25 mg metoprolol) twice a day.
- He also given by some doctors ramipril 10 mg od. If doubt of LVF or frank CCF.
- Every patient is put on statin (atorvostatin 20 mg od).
- Diet, light, semisolid, no sugar preparation for diabetic patients. No alcohol in any form.
- In cardiac rehabilitation after MI role of repeated ECG is of paramount importance in detecting various arrhythmia after MI. Patient is ambulant in ward on second day as mentioned in previous discussion of arrhythmias present medical treatment of arrhythmia prolongs life and patient live better quality of life.

Relationship of MI with ECG changes in different regions of LV and RV. It is already given in Table 6.1. The information regarding ECG lead changes and cardiac muscle damage territory and site of block in coronary circulation are correlated (Appendix 6.1).

- Patient discharged on 4th to 5th day with advice to take following medicine at home.
  - Tab atorvostatin 20 mg HS
  - Tab ecospirin 75 mg od
  - Tab clopidogrel 75 mg od or tab ticagrelor 90 mg bd
  - Tab betaloc 25 mg od
  - Tab ramipril 10 mg od
- He should take rest at home for 4 to 6 weeks. Do walking exercise upto ½ hours and gradually increased to 1 hour per day within 2 months.
- Dietician should give detailed diet chart to the patient and advice him/her to take food cooked with non saturated oils like Suffola, Sanola, etc. and to take fat free milk, curd, stop smoking and alcohol intake in any form.
- To report to his doctor in case of any anginal pain, undue fatigue, breathlessness or palpitation.

Safety of Cardiovascular Medication during Pregnancy and Lactation

Safe drugs are: Adenosine, Metoprolol/propranolol, Digoxin, Lidocaine, Carvedilol, Furosemide, Bumetanide, Dopamine, Dobutamine, Norepinephrine, Hydralazine, Unfractioated heparin, Enoxaparin, Labetalol, Nifedipine, Alpha-methyldopa (oral).

Safety with limited data are: Diltiazem, Sotalol, Flecainide, Propafenone, Hydralazine, Artroban, Bivalirudin, Aspirin (low dose), Clopidogrel, Prasugrel, Ticagretor, Alteplase, Streprokinase, Hydralazine, Nitroglycerine, Isosorbide dinitrate, Torsemide, Metolazone, Nitroprusside, Amlodipine, Hydrochlorothiazide, Clonidine, Statin class.

Conflicting data or unknown in lactating mothers: Diltiazem, Sotalol, Carvedilol, Bumetanide, Dopamine, Dobutamine, Norepinephrine, Isosorbide dinitrate, Torsemide, Metolazone, Nitroglycerine, Clonidine, Artroban, Bivalirudin, Prasugrel, Ticagretor, Alteplase, Streprokinase.

Drugs which are contraindicated for use in pregnancy: Atenonol, ACE inhibitors, ARB class, Aldosterone antagonists, Statin class, ERAs (e.g. bosentan).

Appendix 6.1: Coronary Circulation Block Sites

Correlation with coronary artery branches block sites, ECG changes and myocardial infarcted area		
Coronary artery or branch block site	***ECG changes***	***Myocardial infarcted area***
Left main coronary occlusion	ST ↑ in aVR, V_1 ST ↑ in aVR > V_1 ST depression I, II, III, aVL, aVF, V_1–V_6	LV global dyskinesia ↓ Infarct all over the LV ↓ Sudden death (If not tried urgently)
LAD A. Proximal to 1st septal branch and 1st diagonal branch	ST ↑ aVR and aVL ST ↑ V_1> 2 mm V_2, V_3, V_4 ST ↓ II, III, aVF St 150 electric in V_5 and V_6 Infra-Hisian RBBB may develop	LV–Extensive anterior wall MI, V_2–V_6 (Fig. 6.18) LV–anterior MI, V_2–V_5 (Fig. 6.26)
B. **LAD** mid occlusion distal to 1st septal and 1st diagonal branch	ST ↓ aVL ST ↑ III and aVF > III ST ↑ V_1–V_4 No ST ↓ II, III, aVF	LV Anteroseptal (V_1–V_3) MI (Fig. 6.27) Or Anterolateral (I, aVL, V_5, V_6) (Fig. 6.28)
C. Distal LAD	ST ↓ aVR ST ↑ II, III, aVF (highest in II) ST ↑ V_5, V_6	Anterolateral (Fig. 6.28) Or Inferolateral MI (Fig. 6.24)
Left circumflex	ST ↑ II > III ST elevated I or isoelectric ST ↑ in V_5, V_6, aVL Or ST ↓ V_5, V_6, V_7, V_8, V_9	Anterolateral MI (Fig. 6.28) Postwall MI (prominent in V_1 and V_2)
Total RCA block Right coronary artery	ST ↑ III, II, aVF, III > II, ST ↓ I **Proximal block** ST ↑ > 1 mm with T ↑ in V_4R **Distal block** ST isoelectric V_4R with T wave upright V_4R	Inferior wall MI (Fig. 6.30) Inferolateral MI (Fig. 6.24)
RV infarction	ST ↑ V_1, V_3R, V_4R, V_5B, V_6R	Later Q wave appear (Fig. 6.30)
Posterior MI	Tall R wave V_1, V_2, V_3, V_4 with ST segment ↓ in V_2, V_3, V_4 T wave ↓ V_4, flat T wave V_5, V_6	Fig. 6.31a
Acute anterior wall MI presenting with VT	VT was corrected within 40 meter and subsequently treated for acute MI anterior wall MI	ST elevation from V_1 to V_6 He recovered 4 weeks within uneven for course, he was followed up to 2 years, he refused coronary angiography.

CARDIAC ARREST

Definition

- Cardiac arrest is defined as an abrupt loss of cardiac pump function which may be reversible by a prompt intervention, otherwise will lead to death.
- Cardiac arrest may result from one of the following four mechanisms: (1) Ventricular fibrillation (VF, (2) Pulseless ventricular tachycardia (VT), (3) Asystole and (4) Pulseless electrical activity (PEA) (Table 6.2).

Table 6.2: Common causes of cardiac arrest

Ventricular fibrillation	Ventricular asystole
• Myocardial ischaemia or infarction	• Localised failure of conducting tissue
• Electrocution	• Massive myocardial infarction
• Other structural heart diseases	**Pulseless electrical activity (PEA)**
• Hypokalaemia and hyperkalaemia	• Cardiac rupture
• Drugs	• Massive pulmonary embolism

Management (Cardiopulmonary Resuscitation)

- CPR provides artificial ventilation and perfusion to the vital organs, particularly heart and brain until spontaneous cardiopulmonary function is restored.
- It encompasses both basic life support (BLS) and advanced life support (ALS).
- Successful resuscitation following cardiac arrest requires an integrated set of coordinated actions represented by the links in the chain of survival (Table 6.3).

Table 6.3: Links in the chain of survival

Out-of-hospital cardiac arrest	*In-hospital cardiac arrest*
Immediate recognition of cardiac arrest and activation of the emergency response system (ERS)	Early recognition and prevention
Early CPR with an emphasis on chest compressions (BLS)	Activation of emergency response
Rapid defibrillation	Immediate high-quality CPR
Basic and advanced emergency medical services during transport	Rapid defibrillation
Advanced life support (ALS) and postcardiac arrest care	Postcardiac arrest care
Recovery	Recovery

Immediate Recognition and Activation of Emergency Response System

- Early recognition that a cardiac arrest has occurred is the key to survival.
- If a lone rescuer finds an unresponsive adult, he/she should first ensure that the scene is safe.
- Rescuer should then check for a response by tapping the victim on the shoulder and shouting at the victim (Fig. 6.32).

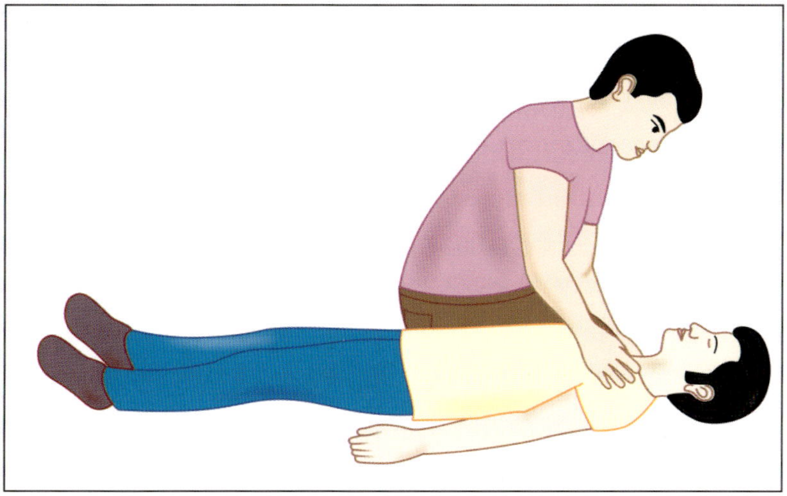

Fig. 6.32: Checking for response

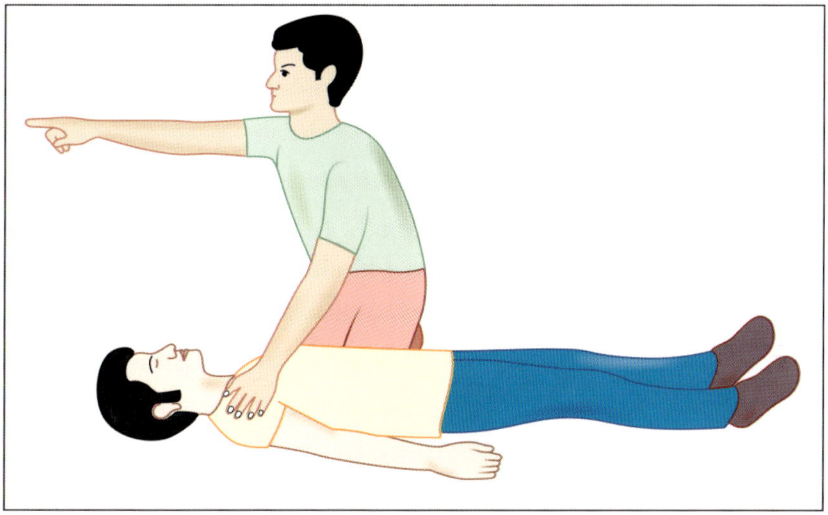

Fig. 6.33: Calling for help and asking other people to activate ERS

- If the victim is unresponsive and has absent or abnormal breathing (i.e. only gasping), the rescuer should assume that the victim is in cardiac arrest. The trained or untrained layperson should activate the ERS.
  - If a lone rescuer is present, he should activate the ERS first and then begin CPR.
  - The healthcare provider can check for a response and look for no breathing or no normal breathing (i.e. only gasping) before activating the ERS.
- After activation of the ERS, all rescuers should immediately begin CPR for adult victims who are unresponsive with no breathing or no normal breathing (only gasping). The rescuer should treat the victim who has occasional gasps as if he/she is not breathing (Fig. 6.33).

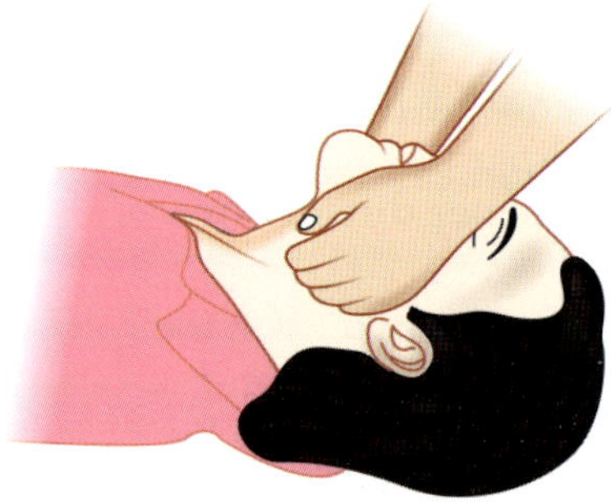

Fig. 6.36: Jaw thrust method

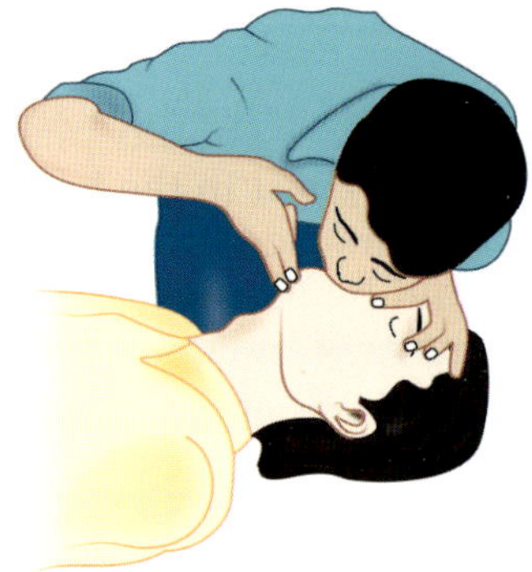

Fig. 6.37: Mouth-to-mouth breathing

breath over 1 second, taking a normal (and not deep) breath. Each rescue breath is delivered over 1 second. If the victim's chest does not rise with the first rescue breath, reposition the head by performing the head-tilt chin-lift again and then give the second rescue breath. Volume of each rescue breath should produce a visible chest rise.

- When an advanced airway (i.e. endotracheal tube or laryngeal mask airway) is in place during CPR, give 1 breath every 6 seconds without attempting to synchronise breaths between compressions; this will result in delivery of 10 breaths/minute. There should be no pause in chest compressions for delivery of ventilations after advanced airway is in place. Tidal volume per breath should be 6 to 7 mL/kg (about 600 mL in adults) (Fig. 6.37).

Early Defibrillation

- Defibrillator should be used as soon as it is available.
- Automated external defibrillators (AEDs) are capable of analysing cardiac rhythm and, if appropriate, advise/deliver an electric countershock. The operator merely places two self-adhesive electrode pads onto the patient and administers a shock when advised, standing clear when the AED is ready to discharge.
- CPR should be started immediately following 1 shock and continued for 5 cycles of 30:2 compression-to-ventilation ratio before rechecking the rhythm.

Basic life support algorithm is shown in Flowchart 6.1.

Advanced Life Support

Advanced life support (ALS) consists of BLS (CAB and early defibrillation) followed by the use of special equipment and drugs for establishing and maintaining effective ventilation and circulation (ABCD, where D stands for defibrillation and for differential diagnoses which include treatable causes of cardiac arrest).

Advanced Airway

6

It includes the use of oral and nasal airways, bag masks, orotracheal, nasotracheal, endotracheal tubes for intubations, laryngeal mask airway and surgical procedures like cricothyrotomy and tracheostomy.

Flowchart 6.1: Adult basic life support algorithm

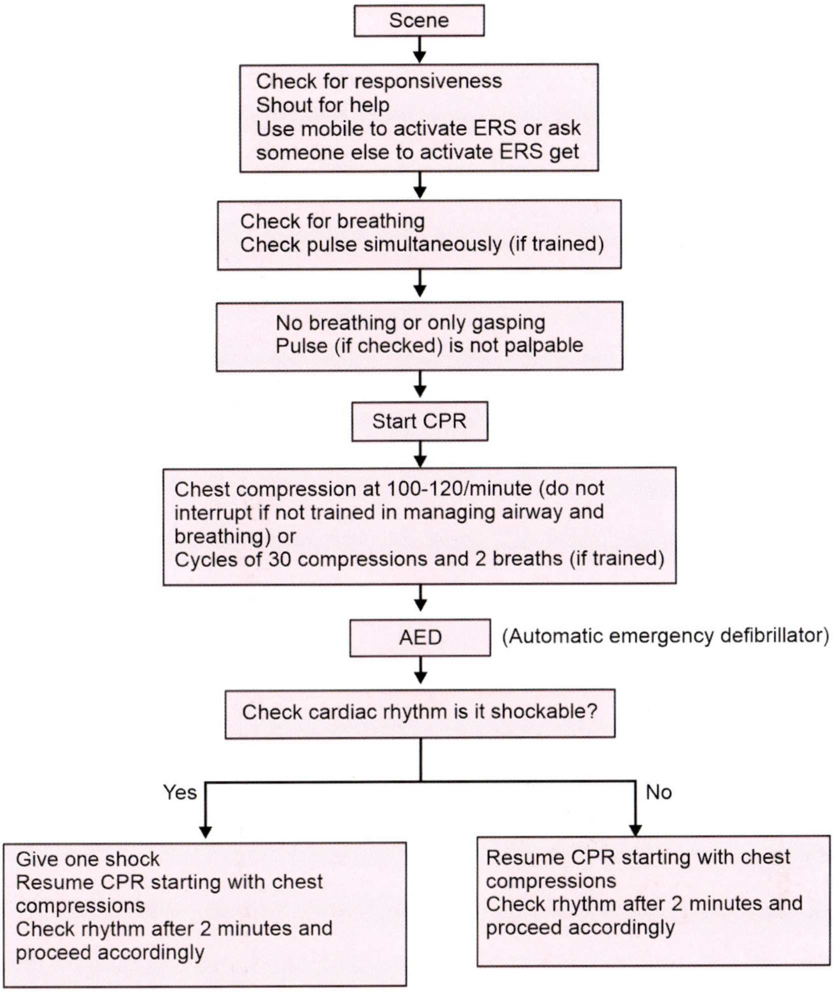

Advanced Breathing

- Confirmation of endotracheal tube placement using both clinical assessments (tube seen passing through vocal cords; five-point auscultation-over epigastrium, left and right anterior chest, and left and right mid-axillary parts of chest; condensation of water vapour inside the tube). End-tidal carbon dioxide is the gold standard to confirm position of the tube in trachea.
- Securing the endotracheal tube using tube holders (which are better than using tape or bandage to hold the tube).
- Ventilate at a tidal volume of 6 to 7 ml/kg and at a rate of 10 breaths/minute.

Advanced Circulation Medical Aid Post/Hospital for in Hospital Cardiac Arrest

- It includes a continuation of chest compression along with establishing intravenous access, attaching a cardiac monitor/defibrillator and assessing the rhythm, defibrillation, and administering drugs appropriate for rhythm and condition.

- With an advanced airway in place, rescuers no longer provide cycles of compression with pauses for ventilation. The compression is done continuously at the rate of 100–120/minute and ventilation is provided at 10 breaths/minute (1 breath every 6 seconds).
- Rhythm checks should be done only after 2 minutes of CPR and not immediately following a defibrillation attempt.

Ventricular Fibrillation or Pulseless Ventricular Tachycardia (Shockable Rhythms)

- As soon as a defibrillator is available, it should be used for early conversion of the fibrillating heart to a normally contracting heart. One shock at 360 J (monophasic defibrillators) or 150–200 J (biphasic defibrillators) is given that is followed by CPR immediately without checking the rhythm or the pulse.
- Continue CPR for 2 minutes, and then pause briefly to check the monitor for rhythm. If VT/VF persists:
  - Give a second shock of the same energy, resume CPR immediately and continue for 2 minutes, and repeat this cycle.
  - Immediately following the second shock, give adrenaline (epinephrine) intravenously in a dose of 1 mg (10 ml of 1:10,000 solution) as an IV bolus followed by a rapid bolus of 20 ml of saline and elevating the arm up.
  - If VT/VF persists, continue giving shocks every 2 minutes.
  - Repeat adrenaline every 3–5 minutes if VT/VF persists.
  - If after two doses of adrenaline VT/VF persists, administer amiodarone 300 mg IV followed by 150 mg after 3–5 minutes if VT/VF persists; start amiodarone infusion (maximum cumulative dose 2.2 g over 24 hours).
  - If amiodarone is not available or is not effective, give lidocaine. The initial dose of lidocaine is 1–1.5 mg/kg IV bolus. If VF or pulseless VT persists, additional doses of 0.5–0.75 mg/kg IV push may be administered at 5 to 10 minutes intervals to a maximum dose of 3 mg/kg.
  - Look for reversible causes if VT/VF persists.
- If organised electrical activity is seen during brief pause in compressions every 2 minutes, check for pulse.
  - If a pulse is present, start post-resuscitation care.
  - If a pulse is not present, continue CPR and switch to a nonshockable rhythm sequence if VT or VF disappears.

Pulseless Electrical Activity and Asystole (Nonshockable Rhythms)

- PEA is defined as cardiac electrical activity in the absence of any palpable pulse. These patients often have some mechanical myocardial contractions but they are too weak to produce a detectable pulse. Asystole is commonly seen in patients of unwitnessed sudden cardiac arrest outside the hospital and in critically ill patients and is nearly always fatal. Both are nonshockable rhythms.
- If the rhythm is PEA or asystole:
  - Continue CPR for 2 minutes before the rhythm check is repeated.
  - Give adrenaline 1 mg IV as soon as feasible.
  - Recheck rhythm after 2 minutes of CPR.

- If PEA or asystole persists, continue CPR, recheck rhythm every 2 minutes, and give adrenaline every 3–5 minutes. Atropine has no role in PEA or asystole.
- If there is a change in rhythm, check for a pulse. If a pulse is present, start post-resuscitation care. If a pulse is absent, continue CPR with rhythm check every 2 minutes and adrenaline every 3–5 minutes.
- In the case of asystole, check that the leads are connected properly and the gain on a monitor is set at maximum.
- If at any time the rhythm develops into VF/VT defibrillate the patient.
- Look for reversible causes that can produce PEA or asystole.

- CPR can be stopped if:
  - VF/VT was eliminated.
  - Advanced airway device placed and position confirmed.
  - Proper oxygenation and ventilation were ensured using an oxygen saturation monitor and end-tidal CO_2 monitor.
  - All rhythm-appropriate drugs were administered.
  - All potentially reversible causes are excluded.
  - CPR was performed for 10 minutes after the rhythm was confirmed to be PEA/asystole.

Miscellaneous Drugs/Equipment in Cardiac Arrest

- Sodium bicarbonate has no benefit when it is administered early during the CPR. In fact, bicarbonate may be detrimental to the patient. It may be used in patients with cardiac arrest related to hyperkalaemia or tricyclic antidepressant poisoning.
- Calcium is recommended only if there is some evidence to suggest hypocalcaemia, hyperkalaemia or calcium channel blocker overdose.
- Fibrinolytic therapy (e.g. streptokinase, tenecteplase) should not be routinely used in cardiac arrest. When pulmonary embolism is presumed or known to be the cause of cardiac arrest, empirical fibrinolytic therapy can be considered.

Adult advanced cardiac life support algorithm is shown in Flowchart 6.2.

When to Stop the Advanced Cardiac Life Support System

When the patient is on Advance CLS for more than 12 hours of its application, and there is no response from the patient either in heart function, breathing, or level of consciousness. Then we have to decide to stop advance CLS, as per the policy of the hospital. Large hospitals have a standing committee of Medical Superintendent, Senior Physician, Senior Cardiologist, and Senior Anaesthetist to decide in such cases whether, brain death has occurred in this patient. To determine brain death following tests have been advised by the British Medical Council.

Tests for Confirming Brain Death

All brainstem reflexes are absent:

a. The pupils are fixed and unreactive to light.
b. The corneal reflexes are absent.
c. The vestibule—ocular reflexes are absent—**there is no eye movement following the injection of 20 ml of ice-cold water into each external auditory meatus in turn.**

Flowchart 6.2: Adult advanced cardiac life support algorithm

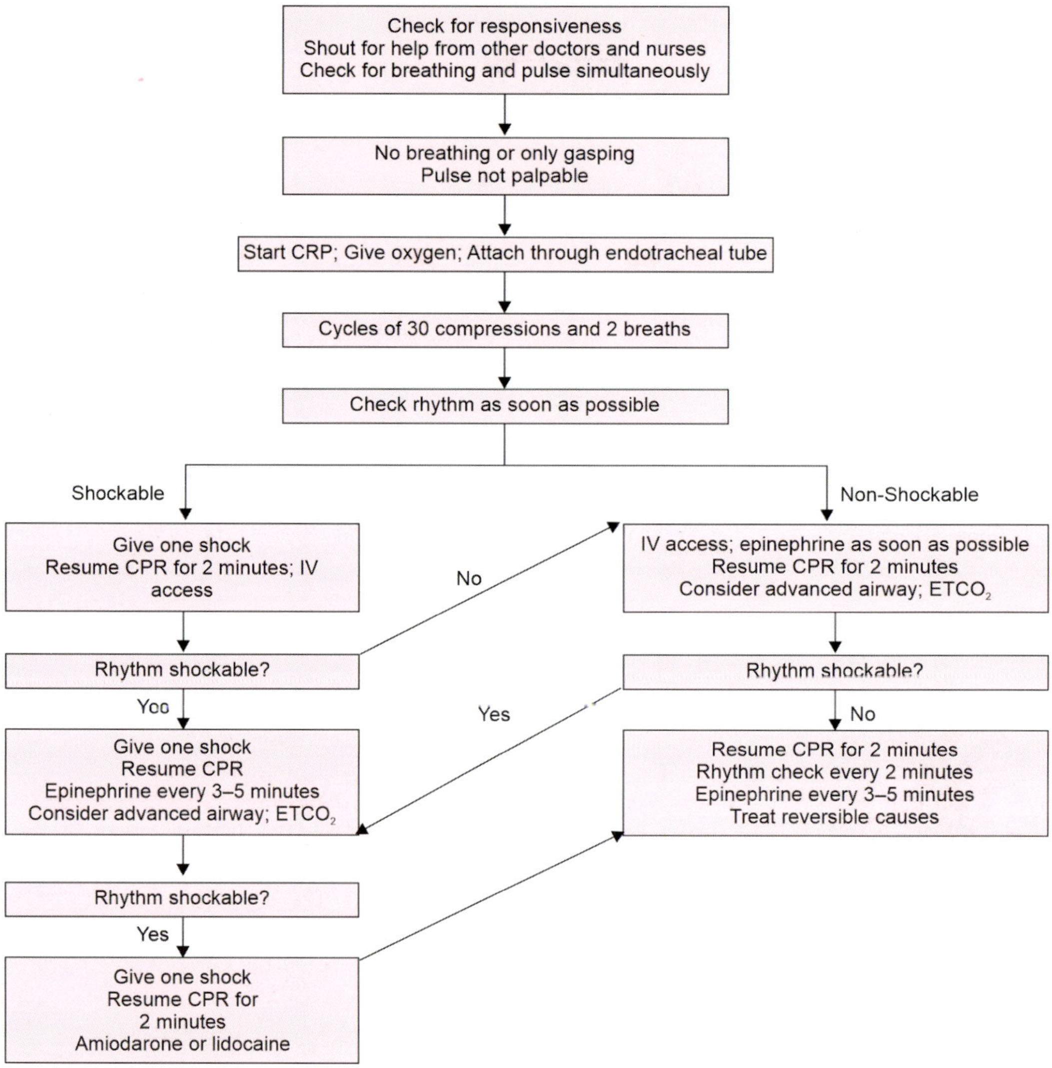

d. There are no motor responses to adequate stimulation within the cranial nerve distribution.
e. There is no gag reflex response to a suction catheter in the trachea.

No respiratory movement occurs when the patient is disconnected from the ventilator for long enough to allow the carbon dioxide tension to rise above the threshold for stimulating respiration ($PaCO_2$ must reach 6.7 kPa/50 mmHg).

If all the test for brain death are positive then in consultation with members of Brain Death Committee, a death certificate is prepared by the residence staff, to be duly signed be Medical Superintendent of the hospital. The members of the hospital organ retrieval committee are contacted by the unit chief of the concerned unit. They will contact the relatives for the organ donation of the deceased patient.

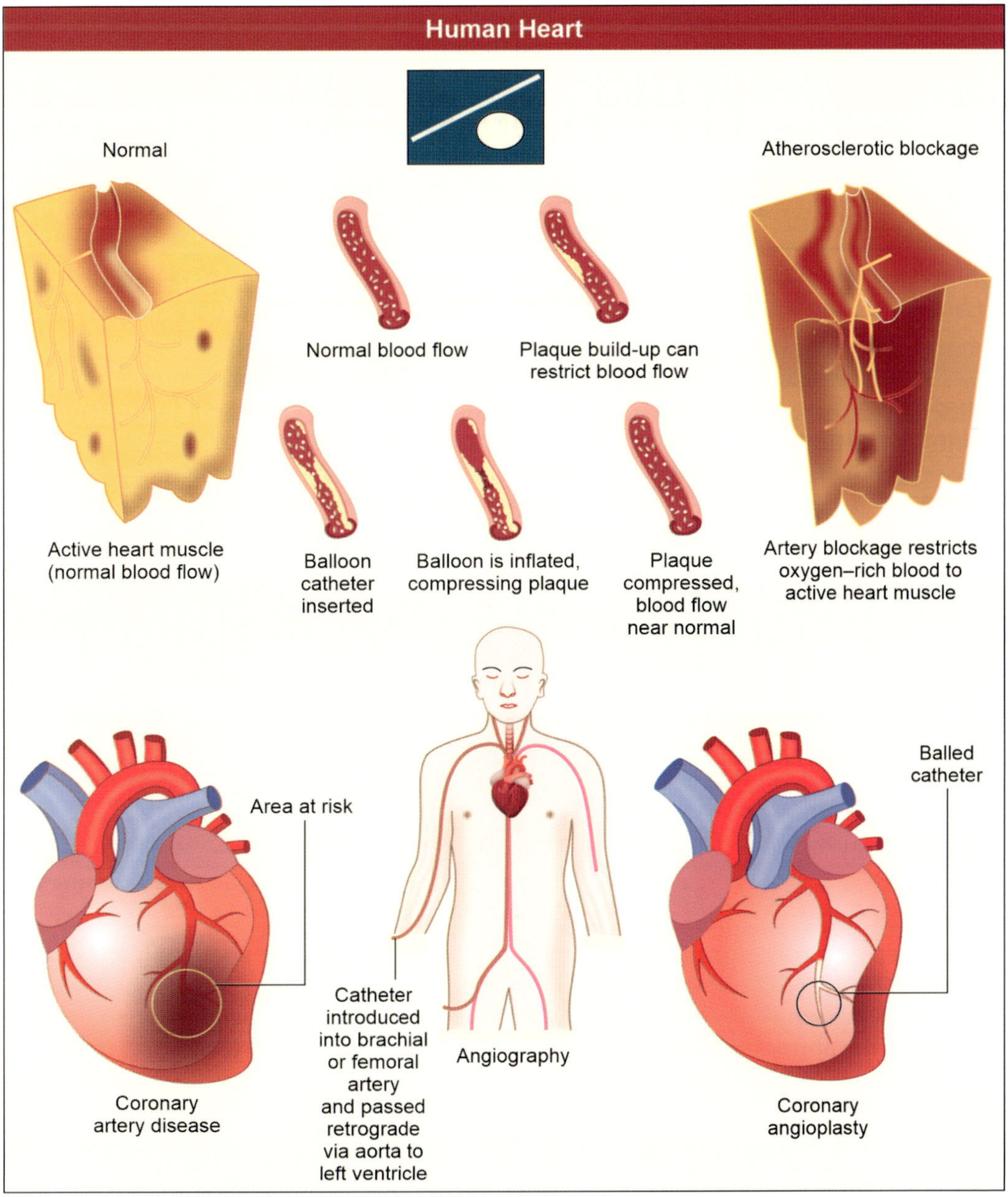

Fig. 6.38: Coronary atherosclerosis from plaque to stent [Progresses very fast in South Asian (Indian people)]

So gentlemen, my young and old friends (consultants of medicine and cardiology), in our country atherosclerosis takes a very heavy toll as illustrated in Fig. 6.38.

6. Selective numbness and wasting of muscles may be seen.
7. Signs of impending or developed gangrene in foot/finger.
8. Raynaud's phenomenon—episodic ischaemia by arterial spasm to cold exposure. There will be blanching and cyanosis of fingers and toes. On rewarming, capillaries and venules dilate and flow rapidly moves in arterioles and capillaries producing reactive hyperaemia. Patient also experiences marked throbbing and painful sensations during a hyperaemic phase.

Causes of arterial disease differ based on the location of the obstruction in the upper/lower limb as shown in Table 7.2 and Fig. 7.2a and b.

Table 7.2: Different causes of PAD in upper and lower limbs

Upper extremity	*Lower extremity*
Atherosclerotic disease	Peripheral arterial disease
Embolic disease	Thromboangiitis obliterans
Subclavian steal syndrome	Raynaud's phenomenon
Thoracic outlet syndrome	Acute arterial occlusion
Takayasu arteritis	Atheroembolism
	Popliteal arterial aneurysm
	Takayasu arteritis of abdominal aorta

Diabetic Foot

In diabetes, a special foot disorder is noted. Platelets have increased expression. Blood coagulability increases. More arterial ischaemia, more atherosclerosis and motor sensory neuropathy occurs. More weight load on the foot, peripheral artery disease (PAD) and microcirculatory disorders cause pressure ulceration and delayed healing. Increased infection is due to poor circulation with inhibition of hyperglycaemia in the immune system (Fig. 7.3a and b).

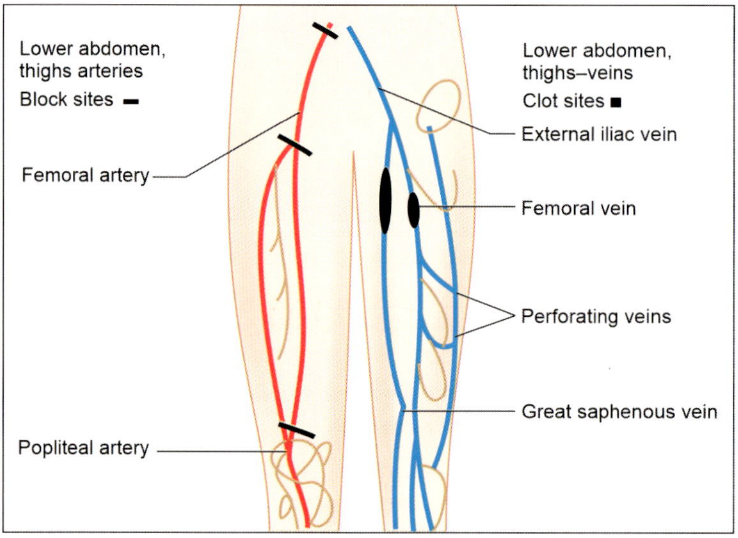

Fig. 7.2a: Arteriovenous system of lower abdomen and thighs

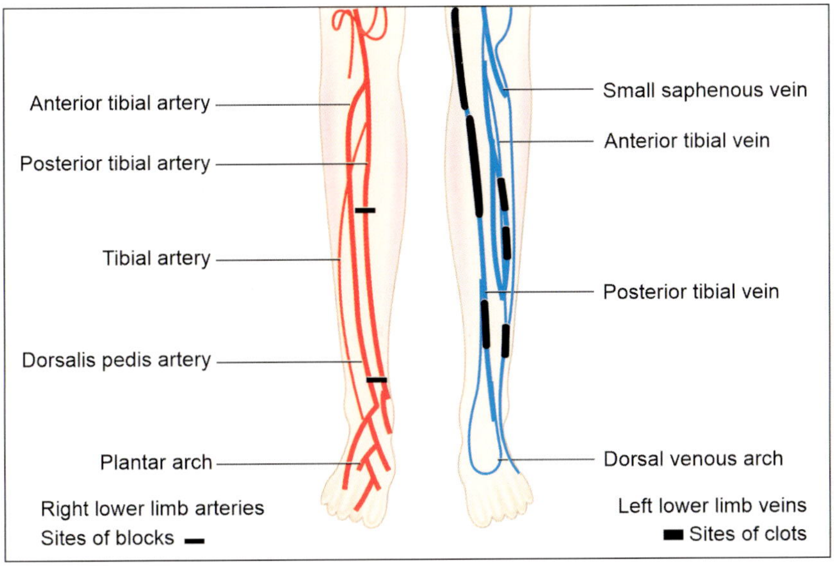

Fig. 7.2b: Arteriovenous system of knees, legs and feet

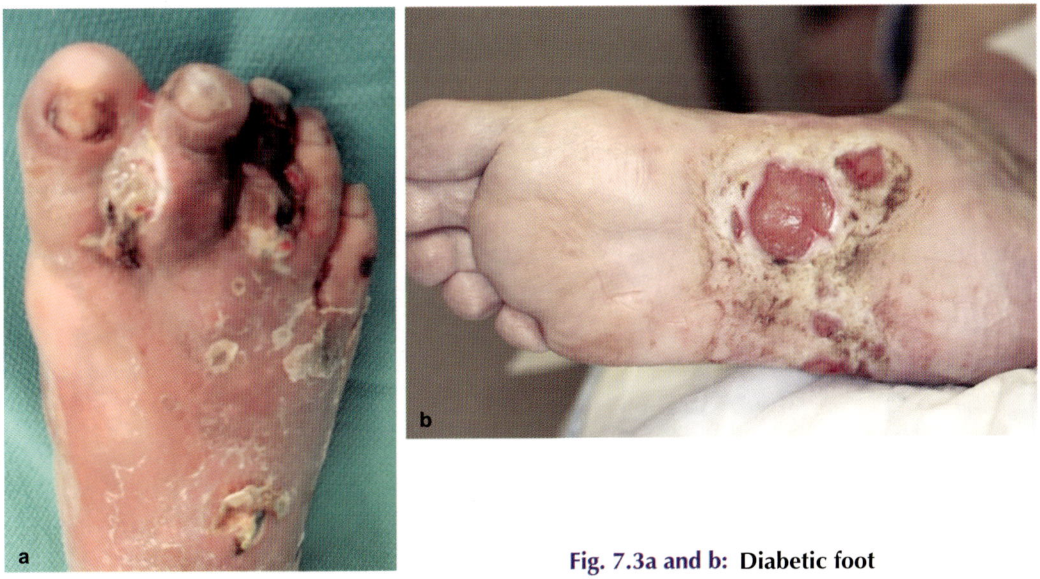

Fig. 7.3a and b: Diabetic foot

Table 7.3: Risk factors for atherosclerotic vascular disease	
Conventional	***Secondary***
Smoking	Hypothyroidism
Diabetes mellitus	Elevated serum fibrinogen level
Dyslipidaemia	
Hypertension	
Obesity	

Venous Disorders in Peripheral Circulation, Particularly in the Lower Limb

1. Compressive—acute deep vein thrombosis and chronic deep vein thrombosis (DVT)
2. Venous reflux—due to defects in the venous valves, e.g. varicose veins
3. Venous compression syndrome, e.g. lonely compression of subclavian vein at outlet by aneurysm or tumour.

Deep vein thrombosis (DVT) is clinically very common and important for medical students and junior clinical house medical staff like interns and house surgeons to detect at the earliest. The most dangerous are embolism arising from it and causing pulmonary embolism which can be fatal if not detected earlier. 40% occur in femoral and iliac veins. The limb swelling and limitation of movements of the limb are observed. Pulmonary embolism patients are dyspnoeic.

In calf veins, deep tenderness felt particularly full flexion of feet. This should be done on all bed patients of major hip joint surgery and chest surgery, who are prone to it. These patients should be given prophylactic anticoagulant treatment.

Varicose Veins

This is seen more in the lower limbs. The superficial veins are dilated and tortuous due to defect in the venous valves causing a back flow of venous blood. Intrinsic weakness of the valves and venous wall may be the cause. Varicose veins are more commonly seen in women.

Lymphoedema (Fig. 7.4)

It results from blockage of the lymphatic system, obstructing adequate lymphatic drainage to the venous system. Swelling occurs, which gradually increases. Primary lymphoedema is due to agenesis or hypoplasia causing obstruction in lymphatic vessels.

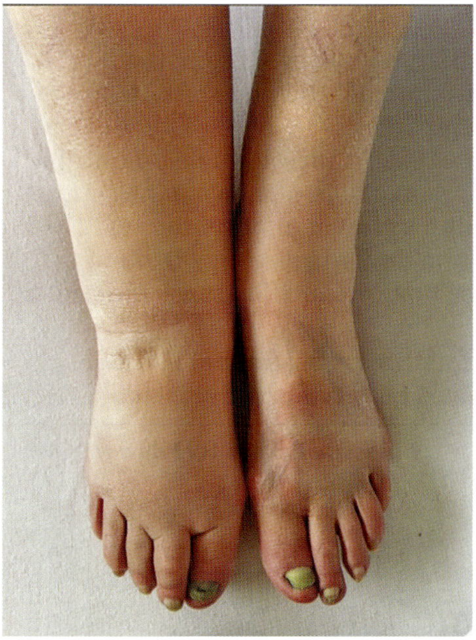

Fig. 7.4: Lymphoedema in right leg and feet

Secondary lymphoedema follows radical surgery in carcinoma of breast. Lymphoedema in the upper limb causes dull, severe pain in the upper limb. Diagnosis is easy. Non-pitting oedema is seen. Asymmetrical swelling of the whole lower limb or foot or leg is also seen. Abdominal and pelvic ultrasound or CT scan can be done to find obstructive cause.

Lymphoscintigraphy and lymphangiography are done to find the cause of microvascular obstruction and differentiate primary from secondary causes. Careful personal hygiene, bandaging of the swollen part aseptically, antibacterial (ciprofloxacin cream) and antifungal (Candid B cream) used when ulcer develops. Lymphatic vessel microsurgery is attempted to open lymph vessels to drain in the vein.

Suggested Reading

1. API Textbook of Medicine, 8th Edition (2010). Published by HQAPI at Mahalaxmi West (Mumbai).
2. Davidson's Principles and Practice of Medicine, 24th Edition–2023. Published by Elsevier, UK.
3. Medicine Prep Manual, 7th Edition, 2023 by K. George Mathews. Published by Relix (India) Pvt Ltd., New Delhi.
4. The ECG in Practice. John R Hampton (International Edition) 2006: Published by Churchill Livingstone, London, UK.
5. JACC – Ageriatric Approach to Percutaneous Coronary Intervention in old patient. JACC Advances Archives Vol.2, No. 5, 2023.
6. 2023 AHA/ACC/ACCP/ASPC/NLA/PCNA Guidelines for the Management of Patients with Chronic Coronary Disease. J.JACC 2023, 04.03.2023.
7. CSI Textbook of Cardiology–The Indian Perspective. Pradip K Deb. JAYPEE. The Health Sciences Publisher, 1st Edition 2018.

Index

J

K

L

M

N

O

P

Q

R